Healthy Body, Happy Life

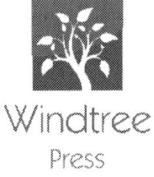

Windtree
Press

Healthy Body, Happy Life

A Non-Diet Lifestyle Guide to Develop a Leaner, Stronger Body
While Avoiding Cancer and Other Diseases

BY MARK REAKSECKER, DMD

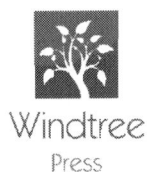

Healthy Body, Happy Life
A Non-Diet Lifestyle Guide to Develop a Leaner, Stronger Body
While Avoiding Cancer and other Diseases

Copyright © Mark Reaksecker, DMD, 2017

ISBN-13: 978-1-94497-341-4 (pbk.)
ISBN-13: 978-1-94497-342-1 (epub)

All rights reserved. No part of this book may be used or reproduced in any manner whatsoever without the express written permission of the author(s), except in the case of brief quotations embodied in critical articles or reviews.

Printed and bound in the U.S.

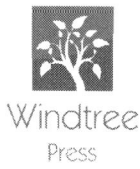

Windtree
Press

818 SW 3rd Avenue, #221-2218
Portland, OR 97204-2405
855-649-0821

This book is dedicated to:

My parents, who introduced me to Christian principles and provided the family model for nurturing and caring love;

My children, who gave me the chance to see this awesome world in which we live through their young and eager lives;

My wife, who has given me the love of a soul mate as we have experienced life's adventures together.

In memory of friends who passed away from cancer:

Gary Dejager

Pastor Gary Ross

Lee Ann Gadilauskas

Linda Palmer

Les Ray

Pastor Wayne Hill

CONTENTS

Prologue

Introduction

Chapter One: The Subject 1

Chapter Two: The Human Body/Food Concepts 21

Chapter Three: Nutritional Supplements, Vitamins and Minerals 99

Chapter Four: Exercise 151

Chapter Five: More Health Hazards 177

Chapter Six: The Garden Of Eden Lifestyle; A Practical Paradigm Shift 203

Chapter Seven: A Look At Common Diseases 253

Epilogue 345

Appendix A 347

Appendix B 352

Appendix C 353

Appendix D 354

Important Disclaimer
Please read!

THIS BOOK CONTAINS information on ways of dealing with health, healthcare, nutrition, diet, various medical conditions, and exercise. However, it is not intended to be a substitute for the diagnosis, advice, and treatment of a healthcare practitioner. Do not use this information in place of a visit, consultation, or the advice of your licensed healthcare provider. Never disregard medical or professional advice, nor should you delay seeking it, because of something you have read in this book. Please ask your physician or other healthcare provider to assist you in understanding the information, or in applying information, that you may glean from this book or other sources.

The purpose of this book is to educate the reader and provide information as part of a general discussion of public health. Medical and health information is constantly changing. Therefore, the information provided in this book should not be considered the most current, complete, or exhaustive.

The Food and Drug Administration has not evaluated any of these statements. Before using any food, supplement, mineral, exercise program, or procedure described herein, each reader should consult with his or her healthcare provider for individual guidance with regard to specific medical conditions and treatments.

Neither the publisher nor the author and editors can be held responsible for any adverse effects or consequences resulting from the use of any information contained herein.

These persons also cannot be held responsible for any errors or omissions in this book.

The author has no affiliation and receives no compensation from any companies mentioned or their products. They are included to provide the reader with a better perspective; the reader is encouraged to further research alternative companies and products. In addition, the references included at the end of each section represent current online sources at the time of this writing. As such, the original formatting was retained. This may appear as different citation styles, but there should be no problem understanding them or the sources of information they provide, whether in these endnotes or the in-text citations.

Prologue

COMMON THEMES PRESENT themselves throughout this book. The general overall theme is two-fold—inflammation is the cause of most diseases, and mitochondrial dysfunction in cells plays an integral role as the result of that inflammatory response, or even the cause itself. These concepts will become apparent in subsequent chapters, but realize that without properly functioning cellular mitochondria—the powerhouse to supply cellular energy—the cells, tissues, and organs eventually die, resulting in disease, including . . . *Cancer*. Therefore, we must bolster our immune system to prevent inflammation and strengthen mitochondria to keep cells functioning at their peak. The best methods to accomplish both are presented in detail in this book.

It took many years to perfect the protocols described in this book, taken from a wide range of sources and carefully reviewed before presenting. Give yourself ample time to acquaint yourself with the procedures. It takes 28 days of continued action to make that action a habit—so be patient. Read this book, practice the suggestions, and reread the book to make sure you are undertaking the activities correctly. Give it all the time you need.

You deserve it.

Introduction

Life is a blessing; live it and share it now.

DIETS DO NOT work. Let me repeat—DIETS DO NOT WORK! "Why?" you may ask. The reason is that traditional dieting methods are too restrictive, hard to maintain, and even downright dangerous to our bodies in some cases. A healthy body requires balance and harmony to maintain psychological, emotional, spiritual, and physical peace. When we disrupt that balance by going to an extreme, such as following a fad diet, the tranquility and well-being of the body is adversely affected.

But what about exercise to counterbalance a poor diet? Sometimes we think we can eat whatever we want and then just exercise the pounds away. Well, that only works to a certain point—to the breaking point—when the shear willpower to maintain that extreme level of exercise dedication can be too much for the body. We then collapse in fatigue and frustration. It is far easier to consume fewer calories than to exercise them off—and, more importantly, it is healthier for you.

Unfortunately, we live and eat in what I refer to as an Advanced Western Civilization Culture. We grow up with a fast-paced lifestyle, eating fast food and sitting countless hours each day at work or in front of the TV at home. This is why obesity has increased markedly, heart disease and strokes are rampant, and cancer is soaring.

Former President Richard Nixon's "war on cancer," which he started forty-plus years ago, has failed. In 1971, one person out of thirty would develop cancer in their lifetime; now it is one in three. Sadly, modern medicine's approach to cancer has not improved the statistics. No magic diet pill exists that will allow you to shed pounds and prevent cancer, all the while eating whatever you want and still allowing you to "look like a model" with a great figure or physique. What, then, is the answer?

Optimal health depends on a proper diet (nutrition, not dieting), exercise (reasonable, but not extreme), and good sleep (plenty of it). The process takes knowledge, discipline, and effort. In life, we never get something for nothing . . . But we can work smart, not hard, and obtain the results we desire. The benefit of this process delivers a leaner, healthy body without hunger, while preventing disease, and especially preventing cancer to the best of our abilities.

A healthy body requires a balance of nutrients at the cellular level and exercise at the muscular level. This requires knowledge of what to eat and how to exercise. The beauty of this, however, does not mean we need to eat terrible-tasting food or exercise until we pass out. We just need to know what healthy foods to consume and which exercise methods are best. It means starting a new life-altering routine—in effect, a paradigm lifestyle shift. It will take determined work since no life-changing process can occur without endeavor. Nevertheless, the results will far outweigh that effort. You will feel more energetic and healthier. I know you can do this!

Are you annoyed with being tired, sick, and/or overweight? Are you annoyed with high blood pressure, soaring prescription costs, and all of the false promises from diet plans? If so, take a quick self-test to assess your health status.

1) Would you like to lose weight, keep it off, and not feel the nagging pangs of hunger?
2) Would you like to obtain a leaner body, flatter stomach, and not feel like exercise is drudgery or overly time-consuming? And would you like to appreciate that working out makes you feel great and want to do more?
3) Would you like to know that you are doing everything possible to ward off cancer and even reverse cancer if you have it?
4) Would you like to improve your self-esteem and feel great with more energy, without consuming dangerous energy drinks?
5) Do you have brain fog, or does it frequently take a long time to get over a cold or flu?

If you have answered yes to any of the above questions, then this book is for you. I will bet that you may have answered most questions in the affirmative, just as I did before I discovered the solution. Let's do this together to get you on the road to a healthy body, happy life. I invite you to come along with me on a journey to get you back to the good health you need and deserve.

To help you think confidently toward this goal, perform a simple exercise. On two pieces of paper write, "I will do what it takes to maintain a healthy body." Place one note on your nightstand so that when you go to bed, you can read it and thereby influence your thoughts as you sleep. Take the other note and place it on the refrigerator so that you will see it in the morning and think about it during the course of the day.

Do this now—I will wait.

Now, each day, read the notes before your day starts and before you retire to bed. Before long, it will become ingrained in your subconscious, and you will succeed!

Let us look back in time to the Garden of Eden, from Biblical readings. As most of us know, Adam and Eve lived in a lush garden with all the imaginable vegetables and fruits they could want to eat. (The Bible alludes to the fact that meat consumption occurred during the time of Noah, as described in Genesis 9:3—"Every moving thing that liveth shall be meat for you; even as the green herb have I given you all things.") Therefore, they were, in essence, what we would today call vegans, getting all their nutrients from fresh food 'right off the vine.' The vegetables and fruits they ate were wholesome and nutritious, grown from clean rainwater and in unpolluted air.

By scientific accounts, ancient humanity did not get cancer. Their existence incorporated fresh vegetables and fruits, clean water, fresh air, less stressful and active lives, and the proper amount of sleep. The Bible claims people lived for centuries. And at the very least, this suggests they lived healthily, long into old age. They lived purposeful lives that required much physical activity including walking anywhere from eight to fifteen miles per day. Furthermore, they did not have luxury items. Ancient conditions sustained a healthy lifestyle that we, as a modern culture, do not experience today.

Modern humans are genetically, physically, and functionally similar to our ancestors. Our bodies have not changed greatly. What *have* changed are the environment and our lifestyle. Today, particularly in the late-20th century and early 21st century world in which we live, humanity is bombarded with adulterated food (processed, genetically modified, and malnutritious), and surrounded by unclean air and water (poisoned by insecticides, herbicides, fungicides, industrial chemicals, and household chemicals). We live with excessive stress, do not get proper exercise, do not get enough sleep, smoke cigarettes, and drink alcohol. It is no wonder we face the current health crises of immense proportion.

In order to correct this ever-expanding detriment to our health, we need a drastic change—NOW!

We must pursue a paradigm lifestyle shift—what I call the Garden of Eden Lifestyle—encompassing a Garden of Eden type diet of nutritious food, if we are to aspire toward healthier living. It can include animal meat for protein or alternate protein sources for vegans and vegetarians.

However, it is so much more than just eating the foods found in the Garden of Eden. It is also avoiding the harsh chemicals present in today's environment, obtaining proper nutrients to sustain us, getting proper exercise and sleep, reducing stress, and eliminating detrimental personal habits. It is a multi-faceted approach to health.

It takes a long time for our bodies to fully form and develop from birth to adulthood, with the brain requiring 25 years for maturation. Just as malnutrition can take years to injure the body from long-term effects, it requires time for the body to heal through positive lifestyle changes. One thing is for sure: if we do not start today to develop a healthy lifestyle, we cannot enjoy a healthier life tomorrow.

There is a wealth of information available on the internet, in books, videos, at seminars, in newsletters, and in brochures. However, how do we know what is sound science-based information and what is simply propaganda? How do we know how to assimilate all the valid information into a practical and useful guide to lead a healthier lifestyle?

This book is the accumulation and assimilation of the wealth of information available from diverse disciplines and seeks to formulate a meaningful solution to the problem of ill health. My purpose for this book, unlike any other book, incorporates all of the pertinent information available to us and provides a total, concise guide to follow. It involves eating the right foods, knowing which supplements enhance nutrition, learning how to exercise, and—best of all—knowing how to prevent, and even reverse, cancer.

Your new lifestyle does not require all-day, strenuous workouts. In addition, you will not feel extreme, gnawing hunger pangs! Would you be interested in trying this life-saving, sane approach to having the healthy body you have always wanted?

Please do not think that it involves sitting on the couch, melting pounds away while eating junk food. There are workout routines that greatly benefit the body, but they are reasonable and practical for everyone—ones that you can do even at ninety years old, and beyond!

The information in each chapter comes from so many sources. It was like putting together an intricate thousand-piece puzzle where the pieces were grabbed from everywhere. They all came together with a precise fit to create something wonderful—the picture of health.

This book entails seven chapters, each one describing topics to give the reader a better appreciation of the need for a lifestyle change.

Chapter One involves "meeting" an actual patient to let you see, as an example, the things that are wrong with our current western lifestyle.

Chapter Two offers a basic primer on the science of the workings of the human body and food-related matters. Its inclusion gives background information on human biology and physiology so you can readily understand the reasoning behind suggestions provided in other parts of this book.

Chapter Three provides detailed background information about vitamins, minerals, and supplements; consult it often as a reference.

Chapter Four discusses the necessity of exercise and includes details about muscle cell biology to help maximize your understanding of the benefits of weight training and aerobic exercise.

Chapter Five offers a list of common health hazards to avoid.

Chapter Six describes the details of the Healthy Body, Happy Life paradigm lifestyle change. It provides methods that demonstrate the positive ways to change one's life. This section will give you a day-by-day, step-by-step, view into a typical week, showing you how all the compiled information guides your personal lifestyle change into a health miracle.

I can tell you absolutely that it has done wonders for me, both in terms of producing physical well-being and the psychological knowledge that I'm doing all I can to prevent disease, heart failure, and cancer. This may not be the elusive fountain of youth, but this lifestyle change is as close as we will ever come to that goal.

Finally, Chapter Seven offers an in-depth discussion of cancer, plus other diseases and conditions, which are all remedied or mitigated by enlisting the concepts of the prior chapters, into a workable plan.

This book was inspired by and written for those who currently have cancer, to give you hope and a direction that offers a better outcome from certain treatment modalities. For those readers not diagnosed with cancer, this work encourages you to do everything possible so you do not have to hear your physician utter that dreaded phrase, "You have cancer."

We need to take care of our own health. Nobody will do that as earnestly as we ourselves will—not food manufacturers, not the FDA (Food and Drug Administration), not the CDC (Centers for Disease Control), not Big Pharma (the popular nickname for the largest pharmaceutical companies), and to a certain extent not even our own healthcare providers. We naturally have our own best interests at heart, so we need to educate our loved ones and ourselves.

The information found in this book will provide you with methods to develop a healthier life. Use this book as a continual reference to consult as needed.

With some topics, there may be too much information to commit to memory. Therefore, if you come across a topic and need a refresher, I recommend that you reread that section. The text also contains words that, for better recognition, have been set in bold print to signify their importance, accompanied by the definition or explanation of that term.

The background information presented is a general guide to help you understand basic scientific principles. The dilemma is to provide background information for a greater understanding of the material while simultaneously preventing readers from feeling overwhelmed by technical, scientific details, especially as found in Chapter Two.

If you are not interested in the scientific details, be assured that by reading the rest of the book (especially Chapter Six), you will have absorbed information that is vital to the success of your new lifestyle.

We are now on the way to giving you the healthy body you desire and deserve, and the ensuing seven chapters that comprise this book describe that process. Along the way, I will explain why each step, plus the applied science, is important.

All right! Let's get going toward creating your healthy body, happy life. We are embarking on a wonderful life-long journey—together!

CHAPTER ONE
The Subject

We've only just begun to learn and understand, because it's all in the course of a lifetime run.

With adversity comes opportunity.

Necessity compels passion and devotion.

LET ME INTRODUCE you to Phil, and his true story. This is not his actual name, but an acronym for Poor Health choices and Illness-causing Lifestyle. He did everything wrong, only to assure he would develop cancer—actually not just one, but two different cancers.

However, let us start from the beginning of his journey.

Phil was born in 1958, in Oregon City, Oregon, to an average middle-class family comprised of a mother, father, two older sisters, and one younger brother. He grew up going to public schools, attending the local church, and playing sports. The standard daily diet for the family consisted of cereal with milk for breakfast, a sandwich and chips for lunch, and a dinner that included red meat with potatoes. But let's not get him started on talking about how horrible was the taste (and how hideous the texture!) of dried, instant, mashed potato flakes—unfortunately one of the new "easy to make" and modern time-saving dinner table staples of 1960s middle-class America. Nevertheless, let's not forget dessert, which was usually scoops of ice cream with all the toppings one could imagine. Phil was quite the experimenter with ice cream toppings and candy-flavored enhancers. If only we had Ben and Jerry's Ice Cream and Cold Stone Creamery then!

In those days, there was not the kind of public concern about nutrition that exists today. Why? Because Americans trusted the FDA to screen, test, and regulate all foods on the American market. Consequently, people assumed that they were eating healthy foods. Dieticians touted the benefits of daily partaking of "the four food groups"—meat, vegetables/fruits, dairy products, and grains/carbohydrates, for optimal health. While the American Heart Association (AHA) suggested eating low-cholesterol foods to avoid atherosclerosis (hardening of the arteries) and the associated heart problems and strokes. So what could go wrong?

Well, Phil had quite the sweet tooth. He loved candy and anything sweet. It was common for him to heap a spoonful of sugar onto the already-too-sweet processed and boxed breakfast cereal. The processed-meat sandwiches he ate for lunch were drenched in tomato ketchup and sweet relish, and the almost daily ice cream desserts often included cake, candy, chocolates, or pie.

Was it any wonder that Phil was chubby? Playing sports as a

child and through high school did not do anything to change that unfortunate fact. Nevertheless, he did try through exercise to regulate his weight.

During his freshman year at Clackamas High School, Phil got a set of weights for Christmas. His thought was to bulk-up his scrawny muscles and eliminate his increasingly chubby tummy. Then he could really impress the girls—testosterone was kicking into full gear. He did some basic study on how to lift weights. He performed the repetitions and completed the sets; but no matter how much he tried, he did not see any real progress. Not really knowing how to weight train correctly, Phil only managed to become frustrated, so he quickly gave up weight training. What he did not know was that results do occur, but only very slowly over time.

When he got his driver's license during his sophomore year, he was able to drive and was off to work after class—at a bakery. As you might guess, that was a recipe for disaster. What is the first thing a growing young man wants to do right after school? Correct . . . eat, eat, and eat some more. His duties at the bakery were to slice the bread that came fresh out of the oven and "ice" the pastry with a white confectionary coating—in other words, to apply a sugar glaze on the Danishes. What happens when you have the combination of a starving male teenager, with a sweet tooth, working after school in a bakery and faced with a seemingly endless supply of ("free"?) fresh baked goods? This was an unfortunate situation for continued weight gain!

Eventually Phil attended nearby Portland State University. His diet had not gotten any better. On top of that, except for some intramural basketball during winter-term, he didn't have much time for exercise. The sedentary college-student life of attending classes and studying at his desk for long hours did not help his health. And talk about the stress of studying and trying to get good grades! No wonder his blood pressure was high—155 over 95, at the ripe old age of 25. An early recipe for disaster, indeed!

After graduating from college and graduate school, Phil tried to combat the inactive lifestyle by playing weekly basketball with "the guys" from high school. Still, that was not enough to stay in shape and sitting for long hours hunched over his work gave him a sore lower back that kept him up at night. It got to the point where he could only sleep about five hours each night. Phil thought that doing abdominal crunches would help; and it did help a little, but not enough. Oh, the aches and pains of getting older—now at the golden age of 30.

Phil's lifestyle did not change much. There was still an unhealthy fast-food diet, little exercise, and no concern for the near future. Until . . . At age 39, Phil noticed blood in his urine. He knew that blood in the stool was somewhat common due to conditions like hemorrhoids, but blood in the urine could be serious. The trip to the urologist to check this out only led to another appointment at the local hospital to perform a pyelogram test.

An intravenous pyelogram test is a radiographic (x-ray) procedure to check for abnormalities in the urinary system: kidneys, ureters, and the bladder. Clinicians found two things of note. One, Phil has two ureters on the left kidney. A ureter is a duct from the kidney to the bladder. This meant that if necessary he could probably donate half of a kidney, complete with the necessary plumbing, to a person in need of a kidney transplant. Two, was that a cyst growing on the wall of his bladder had ruptured, which had caused the blood in his urine. The first finding

CHAPTER ONE | THE SUBJECT

was not so bad; the second finding was not so good.

The urologist surgically removed the cyst and had it biopsied.

It was determined to be a stage one, non-infiltrating papillary transitional cell carcinoma—yes, cancer. Fortunately, for Phil, it was found early, removed entirely, and there was no recurrence of the cancer.

Did this wake Phil up and get him motivated to improve his lifestyle? Unfortunately, it did not. However, in his early forties, he decided it was time to focus on his physical body. College had educated and trained his mind, and now it was finally time to work on improving his body. On the other hand, was this just a mid-life crisis? Either way, he needed to do something before it was too late—so he joined a gym.

Phil went to the gym two-to-three times per week. On Mondays, Wednesdays, and Fridays there was the hour-long aerobics class, after which he hit the machines for weight training. This went on for about five years. There was some muscle gain, but the amount of gain did not seem to be enough for the effort given. Moreover, there was also the fatigue, exhaustion, and drudgery he felt from the extreme workouts. Even though he felt healthier for exercising, and despite the fact that his lower back was feeling somewhat better than before, he became disillusioned with the whole process of this kind of exercise regimen.

During this time, Phil complained of many symptoms. He had high blood pressure, a mental sluggishness, and frequent headaches—four to five per week, requiring painkillers. Acid reflux was another common ailment that required overuse of antacids. Postnasal drip (requiring frequent clearing of his throat), routine sniffles during winter months, heart arrhythmias (sometimes called heart flutter), intestinal cramping, kidney stones, and sharp instantaneous headaches lasting no more than a second were all occasional occurrences, and definitely not fun to endure. Then there was the constant neck and upper back strain along with lower back pain. He also had an unrelenting fungal infection on his left big toe, and he was always tired. You would think that after all the exercise and fitness activity, some of these symptoms would have disappeared. However, sadly, they did not. They only got worse.

It was not long after this that Phil began to develop another symptom. This one involved an unrelenting itch above his left ear. He would continually scratch his head to the chagrin of his wife, who insisted he see a physician about it. (Fortunately for men, wives usually keep their husbands on track to get the medical attention they need.) The problem here, however, was that Phil did not have a primary care physician at the time. In addition, he dragged his feet in trying to find one.

Three months later, in the fall of 2010, Phil finally made an appointment with a primary care physician for an exam. The physician performed the usual new-patient exam, and they discussed the itching above the ear. They surmised it was either a fibrous cyst under the skin, or inflammation/infection of a hair follicle. Phil agreed that if it did not go away, he would see a dermatologist to have it checked.

When it did not go away, it then took six months to find a dermatologist to have it examined. In March of 2011, the dermatologist's physician assistant performed the exam, gave a steroid injection to reduce the itching, and removed tissue for biopsy. The preliminary diagnosis was a sebaceous cyst (a cyst of the oil gland around the hair follicle in the skin). The biopsy

CHAPTER ONE | THE SUBJECT

procedure was superficial and did not include the deep tissues. A pathologist reviewed the tissue sample. Ten days later the report was back—a benign fibrous cyst; irritated skin tissue from repeated scratching. So all was fine—right?

No . . . The itching persisted.

It only took four months this time for Phil to get an appointment with another dermatologist for a second opinion. On Friday, July 8, 2011, he saw a dermatologist recommended by his hair stylist. After he explained to the new doctor what happened at the earlier visits to the dermatologist and the previous lab results, she took another biopsy. This time the deeper tissues were included for review. It would take ten days for the pathology report.

We will digress a moment here. Phil's pastor, Father John Amsberry at St. Joseph the Worker Catholic Church in Portland, Oregon was fully aware of all his health-related issues and requested that Phil describe his life events to the parish during mass. Father John wanted a real-life story to include in his homily. This provides another perspective on the events affecting Phil's life at the time and serves to reveal how his life changed. Here is the actual presentation given during that mass. Imagine you are sitting in the pew listening.*

It started about one year ago with a little bump above my left ear. The bump, the itching, and my wife's persistence persuaded me to see a primary care physician.

The doctor looked at the bump and said it didn't look serious, but to see a dermatologist if it persisted. It didn't go away, so I went to a dermatologist who biopsied the bump. The lab report came back with a diagnosis of a benign fibrous cyst. That's great news . . . I'm OK.

During the following four months the bump grew twice as large, still itched, and was, on occasion, throbbing. I went to a second dermatologist for a second opinion, who re-biopsied the larger bump.

She called me on Monday, ten days afterwards to tell me the results. The first question she asked was, "Are you in a room where you can talk?" Now that got my attention. She proceeded to tell me that I had melanoma cancer. Now I'm thinking, "I'm going to die a whole lot sooner than I expected." I was afraid for my life for probably the first time ever—I can't take anything for granted anymore.

The dermatologist told me arrangements had been made to see a cancer surgeon on Wednesday. After talking to the surgeon's office staff, a PET scan was scheduled the next day, on Tuesday, to see if the melanoma had metastasized anywhere else. The PET scan proved negative. "Thank you, Lord!"

Wednesday, the oncology surgeon discussed the removal of the cancer to a level as deep as he could go—almost to the skull. We also talked about the removal of the nearest lymph node, and the skin graft to cover the removed tissue area on the scalp.

The next day, Thursday, my wife and I saw a medical oncologist to discuss a possible follow-up study and anti-cancer drugs. Then we talked to the surgeon to finalize details for the surgery the next day.

Friday was surgery day. They removed a three-inch-

CHAPTER ONE | THE SUBJECT

round by a quarter-inch-deep piece of scalp and placed a skin graft from my right thigh onto the site. The closest lymph node was also removed. I made it through the three hour surgery just fine. In fact, I was having a great dream—I was on the beach, lying in the warm sun, sipping a yummy fruit drink . . . Then they woke me up.

Because it was late in the day and the surgery site was a little larger than anticipated, they kept me overnight. You cannot sleep in a hospital room from all the noise and the nurse coming in every three hours to check your pulse and blood pressure, so I did a lot of deep thinking and praying. I ran through all the scenarios of possible outcomes of the cancer, from best to worst.

Various thoughts were, will my wife be ok? Would I quit work? How will the bills get paid if I can't work? Will my kids be ok? Where do I want to travel If the cancer takes my life in a few years? And the list went on.

As I lay in the hospital bed, deep in thought at 3:35 am, I surmised life boils down to two basic conclusions that seem to be the most important. First and foremost, if we don't have faith in God our Father, we have absolutely nothing—no hope, no peace, no future . . . Nothing. My faith gave me an inner strength I didn't know I had; if the worst case scenario happens, I know it will be okay because it's God's will, and He is with me—even to the end.

Second, is that family and friends should be cherished. The gift of fellow brothers and sisters in Christ to share our happiness and sorrows is truly divine and shouldn't be taken lightly. We are called to promote the brotherhood of mankind and love our neighbors as the children of God, our Father.

During that early hour, I also reflected upon a paper from the Urantia Papers collection that I had read prior to this entire situation, which talked about man's salvation. It gave me strength and courage. I will cite a paragraph for you:

> *"As to the chances of mortal survival, let it be made forever clear: All souls of every possible phase of mortal existence will survive provided they manifest willingness to co-operate with their indwelling" God-given spirit "and exhibit a desire to find God and to attain divine perfection, even though these desires be but the first faint flickers of the primitive comprehension of that true light which lights everyone who comes into the world."*

Could it be any easier than that? All we have to do is believe in God, trust his will, and through "paradise ascension" desire to be perfect; as our God is perfect. My faith leads me to believe that our God-given, inner spirit in our soul yearns to be back with God the Father, and we are the caretaker of that spirit for the reunion with God in Paradise.

I got out of the hospital around 1 pm the next day, Saturday. I felt great and had very little pain—well enough to go back to work Monday. We had to wait another ten days for the last biopsy report. It was good news . . . And bad. The lymph nodes did not show any melanoma cancer in them. And the surgeon took out enough peripheral

CHAPTER ONE | THE SUBJECT

tissue from my scalp to get beyond the cancer, but didn't and couldn't go deep enough to get all the cancer. This was anticipated, and radiation treatment was to be the next step. I talked to a radiation physician and we began radiation treatment September 12th. After three weeks of treatment, it has caused the loss of about one inch of hair around the surgical site. I think the lesson here is humility.

The radiation treatment could be totally successful, or it could be a temporary measure to slow the cancer process. At this time, I have no idea as to the final outcome of treatment. But I do know there have been numerous acts of kindness along my journey. My wife has posted my condition on Facebook, and I can't tell you all the prayers that have been said on my behalf, from people I don't know personally. Many people have offered to help us out any way they can, in any way we are in need. The love and compassion from fellow man has been awe-inspiring and deeply heart-felt. I truly feel blessed by the best.

I give God thanks everyday—many times a day, even more so lately—I've so much to be thankful for. I feel more alive now, with joy and peace in my heart, and free from the bondage of death, sin, and fear. We don't know how long we have to live on this earth—make the most of it. Share the love of God with others, promote the brotherhood of mankind, be of service to your neighbor, and know you are truly doing the will of our heavenly Father.

Don't be sad for me. This has been a great personal wake-up call . . . I know where I'm going! No-matter what happens, I've had a great life here on earth and know it will be an even better adventure in heaven. Be glad and rejoice with me.

How sad for those who have no faith and no idea what lies ahead for their eternity. We need to help others know that ultimate peace and love from knowing God. That is our evangelistic mission—our duty.

I don't know what the immediate future holds for me as to the recurrence of the melanoma, but I know full well where I'll be after my life on earth is complete. What does the future hold for each of you? I pray you deepen your faith, re-confirm your baptism as often as possible, get to know our loving Father on a personal level, love and forgive your neighbor.

You are loved.

* The Mass presentation may be viewed at: http://www.youtube.com/watch?v=pz4AqvxxS98 It starts at approximately the five-minute mark.

The biopsy report from the second dermatologist's tissue sample revealed melanoma cancer—but it was a variation, called desmoplastic melanoma. This rare form of melanoma occurs mainly in the head and neck region. It displays deep, infiltrating fibrous tissue. That is why no color changes appeared on the skin, which is more typical of melanoma. It can be difficult to diagnose, and often a superficial biopsy does not go deep enough to remove any underlying desmoplastic melanoma tissue for proper microscopic review.

This type of melanoma does not usually metastasize to other areas, but it can often recur locally as it travels down nerve fibers by invasion of the perineurium (the tissue around the nerve). This

CHAPTER ONE | THE SUBJECT

recurrence process is similar to chicken pox, which later manifests as shingles when the virus travels down the nerve.

After finding out he had cancer, Phil's week was a whirlwind with physician visits and a surgery that consisted of removing the affected tissue, removing lymph nodes to check for migrated cancer, and placing a skin graft from thigh to surgical site.

Unfortunately, there was cancer remaining after the surgery, as determined by the surgical tissue biopsy; but this was expected. Radiation treatment followed, consisting of five visits per week for six weeks, with ninety seconds of the radiation dose per visit. Even after this treatment, no one knew if radiation would be a complete success.

About nine months after the radiation treatment, Phil had an unusual feeling in the middle of the original surgical area. It was a strange, tingling nerve sensation that he felt when he touched or scratched the skin. The tissue also felt a little swollen, and it was slightly red in color. So now, it was back to the dermatologist for another biopsy. Could this be a recurrence?

Another tissue biopsy/pathology lab review discovered that it was indeed a recurrence—desmoplastic melanoma will recur locally and had. So now, it was back to the hospital for removal and one more skin graft. The skin grafts were the most uncomfortable part of the procedure for Phil, who said it felt like getting your skin scraped off by a coarse grinding wheel, giving a painful, burning sensation. It heals very slowly.

The tissues above the ear finally healed from the excision and graft; all seemed good, until . . .

Unfortunately, another bump appeared on the back border of the surgical site, and it too had the strange tingling sensation when scratched. The tingling was probably alteration of nerve perception as the cancer affects the nerve directly while traveling its course.

Phil underwent another biopsy in September 2012, which also showed a recurrence of desmoplastic melanoma. Okay. So now it became clear, the previous surgeries and radiation treatment were not working. What could be done next to treat this aggressive, prolific cancer? Phil also wondered if this was the last possibility: was this the end of the road?

The dermatologist recommended that Phil see the head of the Ear, Nose, and Throat (ENT) Department at the Oregon Health & Science University (OHSU). This ENT physician is one of a few on the west coast who performs a specialized procedure to eradicate this formidable cancer. The procedure involves the removal of suspected skin tissue all the way down to the bone and, in so doing, removes all the cancer; but this leaves no vascular bed on which to place a skin graft that would survive—skin grafts need a blood supply to survive.

To alleviate this dilemma, the surgeon removes the outer layer of the skull bone. This exposes the underlying blood vessels in the middle part of the bone on which to graft the skin tissue.

On November 19, 2012, Phil had the cancer and surrounding tissue removed—it was oval and about four inches by six inches above his left ear. A wound-vac covered the exposed inner bone area. The wound-vac is a plastic sheathing applied over a wound and attached to a vacuum pump to provide a slight suction, which draws out and stimulates the growth of the capillaries for use in a later skin graft.

Phil had the wound-vac in place for 20 days. He was attached to the pump "24/7"—physically, but not emotionally. The whirring noise of the pump made it hard to sleep at night, but he knew it was for a short period.

Finally, it was time to remove the wound-vac and to place a skin graft. To be honest, he was not excited about another skin graft—ouch! Now he waited for primary healing. The bandage removal revealed that 60 percent of the grafting was a success. However, this meant there was still 40 percent exposed bone.

In March of 2013, a second skin graft procedure covered more exposed bone. It was partially successful, as more bone had skin over it; but it was still not totally resolved. The skin graft donor site hurt quite a bit, and Phil was left wondering if he wanted to endure another graft or try something else.

In the meantime, he underwent a PET (Positron Emission Tomography) scan in June. The result was great news: no metastasis, and no cancer in the original site.

Consultation with the ENT physician gave Phil the option of either re-trying the wound-vac/skin graft, or trying a tissue expansion procedure. Since the wound-vac and skin graft procedures were only partially successful—and no fun to endure— Phil considered tissue expansion.

Tissue expansion involves surgically placing an "inflatable balloon" under the scalp. Saline is added to the balloon through an access port just under the skin, over the course of two months to blow it up, thus distending or expanding the overlying tissue. After full inflation, surgical removal of the balloon allows stretching the expanded tissue to cover the target area. Suturing it in place allows the expanded tissue to heal over the defect area. This procedure effectively moves the vascular bed along with the tissue, so there is no concern of providing a new blood supply. Phil, in consultation with his wife, decided to pursue this alternative route.

A further consultation with a facial and reconstructive plastic surgeon came in September of 2013, and soon thereafter two expanders were surgically placed under Phil's scalp. Due to skin fragility from the previous surgeries, and radiated tissue, the first attempt to place the expanders failed. Success for the expander placement required an alternate, more reliable incision site. A second, successful placement procedure occurred in December of 2013. After inflating the expanders to 90 percent capacity within two months, they were surgically removed, and the tissue pulled over to cover the exposed bone. More than half of the exposed bone was now covered—progress! However again, it was not a total success. As you might imagine, enduring pain over this period of now years was a challenge and tested Phil's resilience. This is something that people do not often understand fully about cancer treatments.

Another attempt to expand the scalp occurred in September of 2014. A small tear in the tissue around the expander caused it to fail, again. Phil was frustrated. By then he had a large bald spot on the left side of his head—exposed bone that was not pretty to look at—and he had to wear hats everywhere, something he never particularly liked. The plastic surgeon told him the area needed one year's time for proper healing before being ready to reattempt the procedure in the fall of 2015. Phil was not excited to wait yet another year. This had already gone on long enough!

Phil, with the blessing of his plastic surgeon, decided to consult with a hair transplant specialist. If the expansion had to wait for another year, at least he could get a large portion of the successfully skin-grafted, bald spot covered with hair. The added bonus: he wouldn't need to wear hats!

CHAPTER ONE | THE SUBJECT

A consultation with the hair transplant physician went well, and a surgery date was set for May of 2015. This fascinating procedure took about six hours. The back of the scalp was the donor site of hair follicles for transplanting onto the bald spot just above the ear. After donor tissue removal, four medical assistants dissected out the follicles using microscopes while the surgeon placed holes in the receptacle skin site for each of the 641 follicles. The surgeon then placed the follicles into each hole with a resulting density of 50 follicles per square centimeter, which is about half of the density of normal hair. Nevertheless, when fully grown out, it looks natural. Amazing!

The two-week follow-up visit confirmed the transplanted follicles were growing, and the procedure was a success. Finally, some progress! Now Phil would have to wait until September 2015 for the next step when the plastic surgeon would place the final expander and finish the cosmetic reconstruction.

September 11, 2015 was surgery day for placing the tissue expander, and the procedure went well. The incision took one week to heal. Then every two days afterwards, 15 mL of sterile saline was injected into the expander port to slowly expand the balloon and stretch the tissue. During this time Phil could also see the grafted hair follicles growing in the previous bald spot. More progress—maybe slow—but it was still progress.

One month later, the expander was about half-filled. Phil's wife had the task of injecting the saline into the expander. No doubt she agonized over performing this important task and stressed over possibly hurting her husband from the needle stick. Worse yet, if she missed the port and punctured the expander, this meant the need for premature removal of the expander and starting over with the surgical process. She was amused, however, as she saw the expander slowly grow under Phil's scalp and gave him the nickname High-Hat Harry. Phil chuckled and came back with, "I'm getting taller and smarter" from having a bigger head—only to be reminded by her that after the expander was removed, he would be shorter and dumber. Oh well, at least he would be more handsome—maybe—hopefully. It's helpful to keep a good sense of humor.

Twelve weeks after insertion, the expander was finally full with 500 mL added. This allowed for pulling five centimeters of donor tissue across the scalp to cover the four-centimeter defect. The two-hour surgery went well, and the surgeon was able to get the defect margin aligned with the scalp margin. It would only be a matter of time for healing and hair growth to make the joining scar less visible.

At last, the defect was covered, and hair once again covered Phil's head. He felt complete. Even though he was now five years older and sported more grey hairs, he felt as though he had gotten some of his youth back—and had gained much wisdom in this trying and humbling process.

So, the big question: did all this finally wake Phil up?

Finally, thankfully—YES, IT DID!

Phil decided a lifestyle change was in order. He did not want to face another cancer—two was enough. The writing was on the wall. He had no choice. His lifestyle must change; the reality of premature death from cancer or another disease was too obvious. He had so much life yet to live, and he intended to do everything necessary to protect that time and live fully.

Let us stop here for a moment; there is something I must tell you.

CHAPTER ONE | THE SUBJECT

Phil's name was changed originally to save his identity, not to mention the embarrassment from having made so many poor lifestyle choices.

However, full confession is now in order: I am the subject portrayed above . . . I am Phil.

I had made so many lifestyle mistakes—from poor diet, to inadequate exercise, to avoiding getting immediate health care when needed—thereby allowing my cancer tumor to grow larger than it should have. I wanted to share my life story with you so you, too, could see the blunders that can be made by anyone, even a healthcare professional. The good news is that there are alternatives and cures for the mistakes I have made. You would think that as a healthcare provider I would have known better—and sooner. My story just goes to show that we all make errors in judgment, some of which can be costly to our lives. Thankfully, for me, I was spared.

It did inspire me, however, to perform an in-depth study of cancer and a search for scientifically proven remedies. It also became apparent that other benefits of a healthy lifestyle would result. One huge benefit was a leaner body, without dieting. I became an avid reader, learner, and researcher when I found out that I had the second, more serious, cancer. This perhaps is a compulsion that only those with cancer can understand—from facing the possibility of imminent death, you are desperate to find anything that will heal you. You may in your desperation even become somewhat gullible and vulnerable to false promises in materials you read. The purpose of this book is to provide valuable, practical, science-based information that anyone can use to live a healthier, happier life . . . Free of disease. There are other methods to treat and prevent cancer aside from traditional surgery, chemotherapy, and radiation. I would like to share my knowledge with you.

The moral of my story: Do not put matters off. Delays or inaction could prove serious or possibly even fatal.

References

The Urantia Papers: http://www.urantia.org/urantia-book/read-urantia-book-online.

CHAPTER TWO
The Human Body/Food Concepts

Hippocrates (460-370 BC) stated that natural forces within us are the true healers of disease; and that we are to:

"First, do no harm."

"Let food be thy medicine and medicine be thy food."

Preamble

THE DILEMMA FOR this chapter was to provide a basic science background to describe human biology and physiology and its relation to food, while not overwhelming the reader with technical jargon and details. The better one understands the principles in this chapter, the more one will appreciate the conclusions presented. You may even realize many aha, or wow, moments as I had when researching and compiling this information. However, if a science background is not your forte, remember that procedures described in later chapters can easily be implemented without it—the only difference is that you may not fully understand the reason as to why the protocol was presented. This science information is here for your study if you choose.

Basic Human Cell Biology

THE HUMAN BODY is comprised of organs, tissues, and cells working in harmony to sustain life. The body takes in oxygen through the lungs and food through the mouth, while the blood vessels circulate these nutrients to the cells so they can metabolize them for energy.

Organs have their specific purpose, but the cells of each organ dictate the function. The physical, outward nature of all cells is similar. They have a cell wall for structural support and protection from chemicals or invading organisms. It also serves to filter needed nutrients into the cell.

Inside the wall of each cell is a nucleus containing the **DNA** (deoxyribonucleic acid) that determines the cells' function. DNA consists of many genes that create specific proteins, comprised of amino acids. These amino acids perform particular cellular tasks. For example, the DNA of muscle cells code protein to become muscle fiber required for body movement, while nerve cell DNA codes for the ability to make nerves to stimulate those muscles. Organs differ by the specific proteins manufactured in the cells—mapped out by the cellular DNA—that accounts for the organ's specific function.

The space inside the cell wall, that surrounds the nucleus,

contains water, salts, and proteins—called the **cytosol**. This water environment allows numerous chemical reactions to occur, as well as the transport of various molecules around the cell. The water in the cytoplasm accounts for around 70 percent of the total mass of cells.

There are many other cellular components, but the only other one we need to know about for this book is the **mitochondria**. Most cells have several thousand mitochondria in the cytosol, but some can have as few as one and as many as one hundred thousand, depending upon the cell's function. Mitochondria are the cell's powerhouse or energy production component, providing the cell with chemical energy. They produce 90 percent of the body's energy. The health of the mitochondria determine the overall health of the individual, and failing mitochondria are responsible for accelerated aging, disease, and even cancer.

Typically, the mitochondria perform the final conversion of sugar into **ATP** (Adenosine Tri-Phosphate) and **NADH** (Nicotinamide adenine dinucleotide), with the release of carbon dioxide and water as the by-product. ATP and NADH molecules drive chemical reactions to serve the cell's energy needs and its overall purpose. Cells can also use fats and protein to create energy molecules when sugar is not available, but that metabolic process is not as efficient.

Carbohydrates/Fats/Proteins

MACRONUTRIENTS ARE THREE broad groups of nutrients to sustain our body: carbohydrates, fats, and proteins.
Carbohydrates are water-soluble (they dissolve in water) and are the bodies' primary energy source. Fats do not mix with water,

only other fats, and thus are "fat-soluble." **Fat** is a back-up energy source, and the excess is stored in fat cells. Fat molecules also exist in cell walls.

While most **protein** is water-soluble, some larger molecule proteins are fat-soluble. Proteins carry out vital cell operations, like promoting chemical reactions, replicating DNA, allowing cells to communicate with each other, and transporting various molecules in the blood.

When food sources are scarce, protein becomes the energy source. It is not the preferred method since muscles are sacrificed in the process, which if prolonged, can cause an emaciated appearance.

Protein

PROTEINS ARE LARGE molecules consisting of one or more long chains of amino acids. There are twenty-two standard **amino acids** grouped together because they contain a nitrogen atom. There are nine essential amino acids, not synthesized in the body and must be acquired from food.

Proteins have various functions, which differ due to the amino acid sequence. Genes dictate and code for the specific sequence. The resulting three-dimensional shape of the protein constitutes its function in biological processes. Proteins also have a certain lifespan before being recycled by the cell.

Protein is essential for cells and is involved in many processes, especially metabolism via enzymes. They also provide the matrix to give a cell its shape. In all, they are the second largest component of human cells, tissues, and muscles—second only to water. Protein is also critical to make neurotransmitters, which allow our nerves function properly.

Fats

FATS ARE VITAL to the body as they provide the structural basis for the cell wall in addition to being an energy source. Fat is important for the body to maintain healthy cells, organs, and tissues. Many food nutrients are fat-soluble and need fat for proper absorption.

Fats contain **fatty acids**, which are variable length carbon molecules with an organic acid group. Fats with shorter length fatty acids are usually liquid at room temperature, called oil, while the longer chain fatty acids are solid, and are usually called fat. Please note that the words oils and fats will be used interchangeably but suggest the same meaning.

Unsaturated Fats

FAT CAN BE labeled unsaturated, which means it does not have the maximum number of hydrogen atoms that are possible (it has not reached the level of saturation, hence, "unsaturated"). This is due to one or more double bonds existing between carbon atoms.

Effectively, this boils down to the fact that the more unsaturated they are (or the more double bonds they have), the easier the fatty acid can be broken down (oxidized) into smaller chain molecules. Oxidation is one way cells can obtain energy from fat. However, the harmful omega-6 fats, when oxidized, can imbed in the blood vessel wall and cause chronic (long-term) inflammation, leading to **atherosclerosis** (hardening of the arteries due to plaque build-up). We will examine this in detail later.

Trans Fats

WE HAVE ALL heard of trans fats. This defines fatty acids in which the two hydrogen atoms are structurally on opposite sides of–or across from (and hence, "trans")—where the carbon double bond exists. *These trans fats are not found in nature and do not function normally in the human body. They are the result of chemical processing.* Partially hydrogenated animal fats are processed to make cooking oils, but they are harmful in that they are still partially unsaturated (easily oxidized). Trans fats are found in foods that will have written on the ingredient list, "contains partially hydrogenated oils," even though the front label may say no trans fats.

This unnatural trans configuration form interferes with cell membrane and enzyme function due to its angular molecular structure. This makes cell membranes stiff and unable to transfer essential nutrients inside the cell. *Over time, this leads to calcification of the arteries because the trans fats increase the movement of calcium into the blood vessel cells, which causes atherosclerosis.*

Trans fats also interfere with insulin-binding to result in less sugar uptake by the cells, higher blood sugar levels, and the worsening of diabetes via insulin resistance. This leads to more **free radicals** (caustic molecules that oxidize, chemically change and "damage" other molecules) and **lipid peroxidation** (the oxidative breakdown of fat into harmful inflammatory agents). The result is atherosclerosis and higher risk of heart attacks/strokes.

CHAPTER TWO | THE HUMAN BODY

Since all cell walls contain fat molecules, peroxidation or breakdown of the cell wall leads to cell damage and inflammation.

In nature, the classification for fats is according to the length of their carbon chain. They are short, medium, or long chain fats. Short chain fats have less than six carbons, and they contain fewer calories. These are healthy oils for the brain and GI (gastrointestinal) tract. An example is butyric acid, a four-carbon chain that feeds the cells lining the gut and promotes better health.

Medium chain fats, or <u>m</u>edium <u>c</u>hain <u>t</u>riglycerides (MCT oil), have 6 to 12 carbons, and like the short chain fats, are used for energy production. Examples are coconut oil and palm kernel oil. MCT oil is a good source for energy in "**ketogenic diets**" where healthy fats replace sugar for the primary energy source. They also reduce inflammation, reduce cancer growth, and protect the brain.

The Ketogenic diet is a high healthy fat, moderate protein, and low carbohydrate diet. This composition of food induces the body to utilize fats as the primary energy source instead of carbohydrates. Here, the liver converts fat into fatty acids and ketone bodies—hence the name ketogenic diet. Ketone bodies refer to three related compounds produced in the liver by fat metabolism: acetone, acetoacetic acid, and beta-hydroxybutyric acid. These ketone bodies circulate in the blood, pass the **blood-brain barrier**, and are an energy source for the brain. The blood-brain barrier is a highly selective, protective measure that separates circulating blood from the brain's extracellular fluid. It only allows passage of specific molecules from one side to the other.

Long chain fats have 14 to 24 carbons and are the predominant fat found in most foods. Oleic acid, an 18-carbon chain fatty acid, is a very healthy oil found in olives that is mono-unsaturated (harder to oxidize); it reduces inflammation and lowers the risk of atherosclerosis. However, most long chain fats are the unhealthy omega-6 oils.

Omega-6 oils are the "bad" fats that have a double bond at the number six carbon position from the tail end of the carbon chain. They readily oxidize into inflammatory agents in the body. The omega-6 polyunsaturated oils exposed to air can oxidize on your food plate even before you eat them; heat also oxidizes them. Many are eaten in fast-food restaurants that serve deep fried foods in omega-6 oils where the oils are heated all day and not changed often, if at all. Keep oils in airtight containers and refrigerate them to prevent rancidity. These omega -6 oils originate from safflower, sunflower, canola, corn, peanut, and soy. They are the primary fats in processed foods and salad dressing.

The good long-chain fats are the **omega-3 oils**, which have a double bond at the third carbon from the tail end of the carbon chain. Three main omega-3 oils are alpha linolenic acid (ALA), found in flaxseed; Eicosapentaenoic acid (EPA), and Docosahexaenoic acid (DHA), found in fish oil. These are important for metabolism and DHA is good brain anti-inflammatory oil. The problem is that we do not synthesize these well in the body, and as we age, it gets worse. DHA has the longest fatty acid chain and is the hardest and most inefficient for the body to make; thus, diet is the best source. EPA is necessary for the body, but it can also inhibit the immune system, so the better oil from fish is DHA.

The typical American diet delivers a ratio of omega-6 fats to omega-3 fats on an average of 16 to 1. The **essential fatty-acid profile test** is a simple blood test to measure the amount of various fats in the body and can deliver this ratio. Since this is an average ratio, many people have omega-6 fatty acid diets that fall into a range much greater than 16. This is highly inflammatory to our body. For a healthy body, we need the omega-6 to omega-3 ratio to be 5 to 1, or better yet, less. As a comparison, the typical Garden of Eden vegetables/fruits diet, for omega-6 to omega-3 fats ratio, would have been around 1 to 1. It would be even better if the omega-3 fats levels were higher than that of the omega-6 fats. The healthy fats to eat are extra virgin olive oil, coconut oil, omega-3 fats (DHA, flaxseed), conjugated linoleic acid (CLA), and gamma linoleic acid (GLA).

Fat, which needs a place to be stored in the body, is located in two convenient areas—in the subcutaneous fat layer just under the skin, and in the abdomen's **visceral fat** layer. The visceral abdominal fat is the layer of fat cells that surround the abdominal organs, especially the intestines. It is inside your abdominal muscles, not the layer just under the skin. This layer is vital for absorption of nutrients from the intestines, but excessive visceral fat can lead to chronic inflammation in the body.

The visceral fat deposited around the abdominal organs is a store of energy for later use, but they also create another problem. Excessive visceral fat cells also release **cytokines**—which are cell-signaling proteins—that induce various responses from other cells. There are thousands of cytokines, but the ones we are concerned about here are the **inflammatory cytokines**, which stimulate the immune system and cause chronic inflammation.

We need to control visceral fat to reduce the chronic inflammation which will otherwise create many diseases: heart failure and strokes from atherosclerosis, metabolic syndrome, neurodegenerative diseases (Alzheimer's and Parkinson's), and cancer. **Metabolic syndrome** is a condition that involves the association of diabetes, high blood pressure, obesity, and high blood levels of fatty acids, all of which relate to insulin resistance and its effect on metabolism.

We can significantly reduce the visceral fat layer by eliminating all refined sugar, eating low glycemic carbohydrates (discussed shortly), while including healthy omega-3 fats and oils. The great news is that we can accomplish this without feeling intense hunger pangs. Later, you will see how this is possible.

Also, realize that fat cells store toxins: mercury, aluminum, pesticides, herbicides, fungicides, and industrial chemicals. When cattle are fed grass treated with chemicals, and injected with hormones, the poisons get absorbed into their fat cells. When we eat the beef along with the fat, we absorb the poisons into our own fat cells. These toxic materials release over time into our body, slowly killing us. This is good reason to make efforts to reduce abdominal fat and to eat organic meats!

Carbohydrates

CARBOHYDRATES CAN BE either simple or complex—that is, defined by either one or two single-sugar molecules or a complex long chain of repeating, single sugars. The simple carbohydrates consist of a single sugar molecule like glucose or fructose. Two single sugar molecules can bind together—such as table sugar, which is the combination of glucose and fructose—and is a simple sugar as well. It is the special chemical structural arrangement of the molecules and the components that allow for rapid oxidation (metabolism) of the carbohydrate to supply quick energy within the cells.

Simple carbohydrates are not so healthy because they are fast acting, cause a rapid rise in blood insulin levels, and will not satisfy hunger.

Examples of foods containing simple carbohydrates are candy, cake, cookies, pastry, soda pop, and sweetened juices. To reduce the effects of simple sugars on the body, eat them last during a meal so the other foods can dilute and slow their absorption into the blood.

Complex carbohydrates are multiple single-sugar units combined to form very long chains. Examples are starch and cellulose (fiber). Starch consists of many glucose units produced by most plants as a means to store energy for later plant use. Examples are potatoes, wheat, corn, and rice. When we eat starch, it is slowly broken down into simple sugar units of glucose and then metabolized in the cell mitochondria. It can take longer to obtain a rise in blood sugar, so complex sugars are generally considered healthier.

Interesting fact: Excess glucose can be stored in your liver as glycogen and released later, when your body needs it. However, the storage of glycogen in the liver is limited. Once your liver has reached the maximum, your body turns the extra carbohydrate into fat and stores it as visceral fat and love handles—oh, joy.

Cellulose, or fiber, is comprised of long sugar chains that form the structural component of plant cell walls. This roughage is the part of the plant our body cannot digest or absorb. Cows can digest roughage by chewing (and re-chewing) their cud, but it takes a very long time and strong jaw muscles. Remember: fiber is the tree material used to make paper and cardboard!

Glycemic Index (GI) is a term used to index or rank carbohydrates numerically, based on their rate of glycemic response (i.e., their conversion into glucose within the human body). Glycemic Index uses a scale of 0 to 100, with higher values given to foods that cause the most rapid rise in blood sugar. Pure glucose serves as a reference point, and given a Glycemic Index (GI) of 100. It only reflects the available carbohydrate level in the specific food, even though it may also contain fat or protein. It is generally true that simple sugars cause a rapid and immediate rise in blood sugar while complex carbohydrates digest slowly and cause a slow rise in blood sugar. However, some starchy foods, like potatoes or white bread, score higher than honey or table sugar. *Glycemic Indexes of 55 or below are considered low and those 70 and above are considered high.*

The Glycemic Index of food and this other factor leads to an increase in blood sugar. Equally important is the amount of a particular food that you consume. The concept of Glycemic Index, combined with the measure of the total amount of sugar taken in from the food, is referred to as **Glycemic Load** (GL). This total amount of sugar or "load" will be absorbed into the blood from eating a carbohydrate. Also, remember it is portion related—the more portions you eat, the more the glycemic load.

Although most candy has a relatively high Glycemic Index, eating a single piece of candy will result in a relatively small glycemic response. This is because your body's glycemic response is dependent on both the type AND the amount of carbohydrate consumed. *Glycemic Loads (GL's) of 10 or below are considered low, while 20 or above are considered high.*

Let us look at a few examples. Any food can easily be evaluated for its GI or GL from calculators on the internet. Type in "the Glycemic Load for (the food name)." Let us look up average white rice. Depending on the web site, you may get different, but relatively close, results. One site says average white rice has a GI of 89 and a GL of 43. Therefore, white rice has both a high GI and a high GL. For this reason, you would want to minimize consuming white rice.

Some foods can have a high GL even though it has a low GI. An example is vanilla cake packet-mix with vanilla frosting—GI of 42 (low) with a GL of 24 (high).

So which is more important, GI or GL?

The GL is a better indicator for which foods to avoid—if it has a high GL, even small amounts of that food can significantly raise your blood sugar. If you eat high GI foods with a low GL, just do not eat very much of them and your blood sugar levels will not rise greatly. When selecting your favorite foods to eat, it is wise to consider the low Glycemic Index and low Glycemic Load foods. The concept behind the Glycemic Index and Glycemic Load is to minimize insulin-related problems, by identifying and avoiding foods that have the greatest effect on your blood sugar.

Your body performs best when your blood sugar remains relatively constant. If your blood sugar drops too low, you become lethargic and experience increased hunger. In addition, if it goes too high, your brain signals the pancreas to secrete more insulin, which brings your blood sugar back down by converting the excess sugar to stored fat. Moreover, the greater the rate of increase in your blood sugar, the more chance that your body will release an excess amount of insulin and thereby drive your blood sugar back down too low.

Therefore, when you eat foods that cause a large and rapid glycemic response, you may feel an initial elevation in energy and mood as your blood sugar rises. However, following this is a sequence of increased fat storage, lethargy, and then more hunger.

Upon consuming more sugar due to increased hunger, the cycle repeats itself on . . . And on . . . And on. This is how weight gain occurs from eating refined sugars.

Although increased fat storage is bad enough, people with diabetes have an even worse problem. Their body's inability to secrete or process insulin causes their blood sugar to rise too high, leading to a host of additional medical problems, like metabolic syndrome.

Insulin

INSULIN IS A hormone that helps regulate blood sugar levels by promoting absorption of glucose into insulin-dependent tissues, mainly the muscle cells. High insulin levels also drive more glucose to be stored as fatty acids in the subcutaneous (the layer just under the skin) and visceral abdominal fat areas. This storage area is a depot for later use when food sources are scarce.

It is important to regulate blood sugar levels. Deficiencies or excesses of insulin production, can spike sugar levels, or send them plummeting.

Since the brain requires about 25 percent of the body's energy, and its primary fuel source is glucose, one can see that regulation of insulin and blood sugar is critical. If you have experienced frequent headaches from low brain blood sugar levels, then you know the importance of constant insulin regulation.

The body utilizes four underlying secrets to develop a leaner, stronger body while avoiding cancer and other diseases. **The First Secret** is to regulate and maintain *steady* blood sugar levels in a low to moderate range, so excess sugar is not stored as fat but rather burned in muscle tissue. High blood sugar increases insulin levels and promotes the storage of excess sugar as fat; after which lowers the amount of blood sugar. This induces lower insulin production that triggers increased appetite to increase blood sugar levels to protect the brain. It is a vicious cycle.

One way to moderate blood sugar is limit sugar consumption. With less sugar consumed, less insulin will be required to maintain a balance, and the body will be in equilibrium. Another method is exercise; it promotes insulin sensitivity to improve glucose absorption into muscle cells. In addition, a ketogenic diet promoting short and medium chain fats will maintain an insulin steady state while adequately supplying the brain with fuel.

Note: we will see the second and third secret to obtain and maintain a leaner body tone later in this section, and the fourth secret in Chapter Four.

Two other hormones that affect insulin levels and work in opposing fashion are ghrelin and leptin. **Ghrelin** is the "hunger hormone" released from the gastrointestinal tract (GI) when the brain senses a lack of sugar to feed the brain, which induces the desire to eat. This hormone releases, after a plummet of blood sugar, to decrease the insulin levels and raise blood sugar levels. **Leptin** has just the opposite effect and is the "satiation hormone" that signals when the body is nutrient-satisfied. When we get enough nutrients, and the blood sugar levels are higher, the hormone kicks in to stimulate insulin first to drive glucose into cells for metabolism, and then to store excesses in fat cells for later use. This intense high and low blood-insulin pattern needs regulation so steady burning of sugar occurs and the body is not storing sugar as fat.

Another important hormone that helps regulate metabolism is

adiponectin, a protein that signals the body to oxidize fat for fuel. The more adiponectin circulating in the blood, the more fat burned in metabolism. It is produced in fat tissues; but counter-intuitively, the more fat one has, the less it is secreted. This is why obese people have lower circulating levels of this hormone. Weight reduction reverses this process and significantly increases adiponectin levels in blood.

Adiponectin and leptin are synergistic and their actions complimentary; mice studies have shown these two hormones completely reverse insulin resistance. Thus, more muscle cells take up glucose and burn fat due to these two hormones.

Adiponectin levels in humans are reduced in diabetics compared to non-diabetics—thus more fat is stored because insulin resistance has increased. Increasing adiponectin levels can help Type 2 diabetics and curb appetite. There are foods that promote adiponectin, which will be examined in Chapter Seven when we discuss obesity in greater detail.

Insulin receptor resistance also plays a huge role. **Insulin resistance** will cause the pancreas to generate more blood insulin since the body knows high blood levels are present and not enough glucose absorbs into the cells.

The problem is that no amount of insulin will correct poor functioning insulin receptors—called insulin resistance. With continued high insulin levels, more glucose and fatty acids are stored as fat, while fat itself is prevented from leaving the cells to be used as energy. If there are not enough cells to store fat, more will be created for you—just what you wanted.

Aging causes the muscle cells to be more resistant to insulin and thus less glucose enters the muscle cells to generate energy, while more diverts into the fat cells. This explains why we get weaker and more sedentary with age. We also develop a larger mid-section or beer-belly (in men) and thigh/buttocks (in women). A misconception is that obese people are fat because they are always eating. However, in fact, they are eating because their fat stores are getting most of the food energy, robbing them of satiation. If the muscle-cell insulin receptors were less resistant and more glucose diverted into muscle cells, the process would reverse, and they would become less obese.

The good news is that supplements, proper nutrition, and exercise can remedy this. Aging causes the cell enzymes to react slowly; healthy supplement levels can get them energized again to aid cell repair and boost energy. This can help prevent or reverse insulin dependence in the body and correct obesity.

Reactive Hypoglycemia

FORTY PERCENT OF the US population has **reactive hypoglycemia**. It is a condition where the release of excessive insulin, induced by eating a high glycemic meal, causes a rebound low blood sugar level (hypoglycemia). Insulin, secreted by the pancreas, facilitates the uptake of sugar into muscle, and other tissue cells. The body must maintain a balance between glucose absorption for muscle metabolism, while allowing enough glucose to cross the blood brain barrier to fuel the brain. If there is excess insulin, the muscle tissues will absorb most glucose and there will not be enough blood glucose to supply the brain with energy. This can be dangerous because prolonged untreated episodes can lead to a coma and even death.

Some of the common symptoms of reactive hypoglycemia are

blurred vision, cold or numbness in the extremities, confusion, depression, dizziness, fatigue, headaches, irritability, and panic attacks. Headaches are an early warning sign of glucose deprivation in the brain, and indicate low blood sugar levels. To remedy the headache, fuel the brain with MCT oil, healthy omega-3 fats, and coconut oil. My preference is coconut oil (it contains MCT oil) with some almonds—a healthy snack that fuels the brain.

It is paramount to maintain a steady, level state of blood glucose levels, which simultaneously feeds the muscles, fuels the brain, and helps burn fat stores—the first secret to a leaner body.

Various remedies can alleviate reactive hypoglycemia. One can limit sugar intake directly, eat smaller and more frequent meals, and choose more high fiber foods—these practices help create a blood sugar steady state. Regular exercise will also help increase sugar uptake into muscle cells and deplete excessive insulin released into the blood.

Glucagon is a hormone produced in the pancreas that raises the blood levels of glucose. It has the opposite effect of insulin and increases blood sugar levels. Thus, insulin and glucagon are part of a biofeedback system to regulate glucose at a constant level. When blood levels of glucose are too low, the release of glucagon causes the liver to convert stored glycogen back into glucose in the blood. Therefore, glucagon reverses the effect of reactive hypoglycemia. It also regulates the storage of glucose into fat by inhibiting the process so more glucose will remain in the blood.

Glucose Oxidation for Fuel

LET US LOOK at how sugar (glucose) metabolizes into chemical energy after insulin drives it into cells. Complete oxidation of one glucose molecule converts it into six carbon dioxide and forty-two water molecules, with the production of as many as thirty-six ATP. This process is called the **citric acid cycle**, or **Krebs cycle**, and *it occurs in the mitochondria*. A brief description of this process follows for those who crave the technical chemical jargon.

The first step is **glycolysis** and occurs in the cell cytosol. Here, glucose metabolizes into pyruvate, a three-carbon chain, plus two ATP. This process does not require oxygen and is the **anaerobic** (without oxygen) metabolic phase. From here, one of two processes occurs. Either the pyruvate enters into the mitochondria for oxidation, or if there is a lack of oxygen, the pyruvate ferments into lactic acid in the cytosol. In the case of prolonged muscle contractions through intense activity, oxygen is totally consumed and excess glucose cannot be fully oxidized into carbon dioxide and water. It transforms into two lactic acid molecules and two more ATP. Thus, from fermentation, we only get four ATP; this is highly inefficient and causes muscle and joints to ache from lactic acid buildup.

When the pyruvate molecule transports into the mitochondria with available oxygen, the aerobic phase of cellular metabolism of glucose ensues. Through oxidation of pyruvate, thirty-four more ATP form, for thirty-six total ATP formed from glucose. Here the pyruvate metabolizes through a series of steps, with the use of enzymes, into carbon dioxide. Water forms from a concurrent metabolic process involving NADH.

Fatty acids can also oxidize in the mitochondria, generating ATP chemical energy. The amount of ATP generated depends on the length of the fatty acid carbon chain.

Cholesterol

CHOLESTEROL IS A group of five lipoproteins, which are composed of multiple proteins that transport cholesterol, phospholipids, or triglyceride molecules around the body. This allows the fats to reach the cells and perform their function. The five lipoproteins are chylomicrons (ULDL), very low-density lipoprotein (VLDL), low-density lipoprotein (LDL), intermediate-density lipoprotein (IDL), and high-density lipoprotein (HDL); all are smaller than human cells. The two cholesterol lipoprotein groups people are usually interested in are LDL and HDL.

High-density lipoprotein (good cholesterol) protects against atherosclerosis by removing fat molecules from the wall of arteries. Low-density lipoprotein has two sub-components. The first is the "large-molecule LDL" (like HDL, it is hard to oxidize and is protective). The second is "small-dense LDL" that oxidizes easily and is the only component associated with atherosclerosis. Thus, the only component that matters is small-dense LDL because it is able to transport fat content into artery walls, cause inflammation, and thus drive atherosclerosis.

Cholesterol provides nine important body functions that we must have for survival. It makes cortisol (the stress hormone); sex hormones (estrogen, progesterone, and testosterone); is required for the body to make vitamin D3; and makes bile salts. Cholesterol is also an antioxidant; is used by brain serotonin receptors (vital for proper growth of a baby's brain); helps in the nervous and immune systems; aids proper intestine function (helps prevent leaky gut syndrome) and repairs damaged cell walls. As you can see, cholesterol is very important and is a vital component to our health.

Triglycerides are esters comprised of a glycerol head (a three-carbon chain, each with a hydrogen/oxygen group) and three fatty acid tails. As a blood lipid, it enables the transfer of fat and glucose from the liver to other cells. The fatty acid tails can be the same or different lengths (usually 16, 18, or 20 carbons long), which dictates the various organic molecular properties.

In 1950, Dr. John Gofman, a professor of medical physics at the University of California, discovered that the triglyceride levels are closely linked to atherosclerosis and heart disease. The major regulator of triglyceride levels in the blood, is not cholesterol or fat, but is the consumption of refined sugar and high glycemic carbohydrates.

If you limit these dietary sugars, the triglycerides will be reduced, the LDL will be lower, and the HDL will be higher. Therefore reduce your sugar intake to reduce the triglycerides and reduce risk of inflammation and atherosclerosis—this also helps to regulate insulin levels and ward off hunger.

A more accurate assessment than LDL cholesterol for risk of heart disease and stroke is the ratio of HDL/total cholesterol, multiplied by 100. Here we like to see a high HDL and low total cholesterol so a result greater than 24 is good, while below 10 is high risk. An even better assessment is the triglyceride/HDL ratio. We want to see a low triglyceride level and high HDL cholesterol.

As seen above, the triglycerides are a better indicator of the level of inflammation and are very dependent upon sugar consumption. A triglyceride/HDL ratio value Less than 2 signifies low risk for heart disease and stroke.

The reason triglyceride levels are a better indicator is that they are directly associated with inflammation. Higher triglyceride levels equal more inflammation. For cholesterol to produce inflammation, it must be oxidized to create a free radical. A free radical is an especially reactive atom or molecule that can damage cells, proteins, and DNA by altering their chemical structure. Un-oxidized LDL cholesterol is harmless. If your diet includes plenty of **antioxidants** (atoms or molecules that render free radicals harmless), only minute amounts of oxidized cholesterol will result.

When Dr. Gofman performed his research, he found *triglycerides* in the atherosclerotic plaque within the arteries. However, the inflammation was attributed to cholesterol by other researchers. *We now know that processed sugar is harmful and omega-3 fats are healthy.* This also explains why diabetics, who often have normal or low levels of cholesterol, have such a high incidence of heart disease and stroke. Moreover, remember cholesterol is a vital lipoprotein that the body must have to survive—low levels are detrimental to proper biological function.

Sugar, which is found in many foods and soda pop, especially HFCS (high fructose corn syrup), greatly enhances inflammation by promoting insulin resistance which keeps blood sugar levels high. This promotes free radical production, which leads to inflammation and atherosclerosis, thus increasing the risk for hypertension, cardiovascular disease, and cancer.

Statin Drugs

STATIN DRUGS MAY reduce cholesterol, but they have numerous serious side effects. One is the depletion of the body's essential energy-stimulating molecule CoQ10 that aids cellular mitochondria to produce energy. The lack of CoQ10 can lead to congestive heart failure by slowly killing heart-muscle cells. Also seen is extreme muscle weakness and breakdown of muscle fibers—it is hard to build muscle bulk while taking statin drugs. Other side effects are neurological disorders, painful joints, dementia-like memory loss, irritability, death, suppression of the immune system cells that can lead to cancer, and to fungal, viral, and bacterial infections. Do any these side effects sound appealing?

An article written in The Express (www.express.co.uk/lifestyle/health/608210/statins-age-you-faster-new-research-suggests-long-term-use-warning) discusses aging as a side effect of statin drugs:

> "Statins make regular users become older faster, leaving them open to long-term mental and physical decline"

The article continues:

> "Scientists have found the heart disease drug badly affects our stem cells, the internal medical system which repairs damage to our bodies and protects us from muscle and joint pain as well as memory loss . . . Professor Reza Izadpanah, a stem cell biologist and lead author of the research published in the American Journal of Physiology, said: "Our study shows statins may speed up the ageing process."

This statement above is important to remember when cancer stem cells are discussed in Chapter Seven.

My healthcare provider wanted me to take a statin drug since my LDL was slightly elevated. I told him that since my HDL/total cholesterol ratio percentage was greater than 24, and my triglyceride/HDL ratio was less than two, I was not worried about atherosclerosis from cholesterol. Rather, I was more worried about dying from heart failure by taking the statin drug. Besides, studies show the benefit of statins to decrease the risk of heart disease of only one person in a hundred, or just one percent—but this says nothing about the harmful side effects from taking the statin drug in the first place.

Also associated with diminished CoQ10 levels from statins is the deficiency of magnesium. Approximately 75 percent of Americans are already magnesium deficient, so why amplify the problem. In case you are wondering, magnesium is beneficial for over 300 enzymatic reactions in the body. So yes, it is a very critical element.

When you test for magnesium levels, have the healthcare provider perform an RBC (red blood cell) essential mineral test. This measures the actual amount of magnesium that is absorbed and utilized by the body, not just the amount floating around in the blood. Just like any other nutrient, if the tissues do not absorb it, magnesium will not be beneficial to the body. Magnesium can also help to lower LDL levels.

Another test to determine the amount of body inflammation is the CRP (C-reactive protein) test. This measures the amount of inflammatory cytokines in the body resulting from inflammation. A result of less than one shows minimal concern for inflammation and atherosclerosis. The only problem with this test is that if the results indicate inflammation, it does not tell you where it is in your body.

It has been shown that statins are ineffective in lowering cholesterol for those older than 65. Thyroid hormone levels diminish with age, and as the thyroid hormone thyroxine decreases, levels of cholesterol increase.

Thus, a better approach is to have your thyroid levels checked and supplement as needed. The thyroid-stimulating hormone (TSH) is commonly tested, but it only demonstrates the amount of TSH produced by the pituitary gland. The effect on the thyroid gland from TSH may be minimal. It is better to test for the actual hormones of T4, the precursor thyroxine hormone, and T3, the functional form of thyroxine. If you are deficient in T3 thyroxine, supplement to increase its level, which simultaneously decreases cholesterol. In addition, it has been shown that 20 mg per day of policosanol can reduce cholesterol levels, without the side effects. Ultimately, the best way to control cholesterol is by diet, through the reduction of refined sugar intake.

Here are a few more notes on statins. They are powerful immune suppressants and mildly anti-inflammatory, so the benefits come from reducing the inflammation, not the cholesterol level. Very low cholesterol levels can be harmful as this increases the chance for brain hemorrhage (and death); and after the age of 70, there is increased risk of dementia. Better options than statin drugs are to reduce the intake of refined sugar, eat healthy omega-3 fats, supplement with antioxidants, magnesium, and CoQ10, and take thyroid hormone T3 if your levels are low.

Google and read the harmful effects of statins. There are numerous studies to prove this claim. One study by the physician Dr. Golomb, found at http://www.ncbi.nlm.nih.gov/pmc/articles/PMC2849981/, describes the damage they cause to mitochondria, the cell's energy factory. Compounding the problem, the abstract declares that prescribers of these dangerous drugs are not fully aware of the side effects. It states, "Physician awareness of statin AEs (adverse effects) is reportedly low even for the AEs most widely reported by patients." We as patients need to read, study, and become informed; this is our personal health and life affected.

Starvation Diets

STARVATION DIETS THAT drastically cut calories across the carbohydrate, protein, and fat macronutrient structure do not work. A starving body will suppress energy usage by decreasing thyroxine levels from the thyroid gland, which lowers metabolism. Then, if you eat a diet full of sugar, this causes a rapid rise in blood insulin levels. While the body thinks it is in energy conservation mode, the insulin will store the glucose and fatty acids in the fat cells; thus, you actually gain fat. This is why you will look heavier even though you may be losing weight. This promotion in the past by food manufacturers to replace fat with cheap but unhealthy sugar has led to undesired results.

    The harmful part of a starvation diet is that once the immediate (glucose) and intermediate (fat) energy sources are no longer available, the body goes after the final energy reserve—it consumes muscle protein, the least efficient energy source. The protein in muscle will be consumed as a last ditch energy source and muscle mass becomes lost. This may also be the reason for weight reduction even though more fat is stored—muscle weighs more than fat. This explains why long distance runners do not look very muscular, they burn muscle protein for energy because the immediate and intermediate fuel sources are exhausted during extensive energy demands.

The Healthy Diet

THE MOST IMPORTANT weapon we have against aging and disease is our diet—it can provide healthy beneficial nutrients, or it can be loaded with harmful, illness and cancer-causing foods. The body likes and needs balance—harmony. We are healthiest when we have balance.

Most people, especially in the U.S., do not understand why we eat — that is, why our brain signals that we are hungry. It is not to impart pleasure. In fact, pleasure is merely a byproduct so you will not neglect to eat altogether. Rather, we eat to supply our bodies with the essential nutrients necessary to function and for protection. Most American diets contain few healthy nutrients along with many damaging substances.

When we talk to others about the food they eat (especially from a restaurant), people often ask, "Was it good?" They want to know if it tasted good, as though, if it tasted good, it was also good for them. However, are we talking the same thing? Often we do not really know if it was good for us, we just hope for the best. That is why we need to know if food is healthy, so we can honestly respond, "Yes, it was good." Many foods can be healthy and taste good, while just as many can taste great and cause cancer from repeated consumption (for example, GMO foods that will be discussed later).

Our diet should consist of a variety of foods that contain all three macronutrients, in proportions that sustain a healthy body. We cannot eliminate fat and eat more sugar, or eat mostly protein and little carbohydrates. Our bodies require a balance; a diet that throws off the harmony will not sustain a healthy body.

The basic macronutrient percentages to sustain normal biological function, according to the Food and Nutrition Board of the Institutes of Medicine (IOM) acceptable macronutrient distribution ranges, are carbohydrates 40-50%, protein 25-35%, and fat 10-30%. These values will adjust up or down, depending on a person's age, sex, and the amount of physical activity they undertake. An easy and approximate ratio to remember for carbohydrates to protein to fat is 2:1:1; or 50% carbohydrates, 25% protein, and 25% fat.

Athletes have slightly higher carbohydrate and protein needs compared to sedentary individuals. Children ages one to three need slightly higher fat percentages to maintain proper initial development. Also, strive to consume less than 2500 mg of sodium as well as more than 25 grams of fiber.

High-protein, low-carbohydrate diets are often effective for weight loss because they can lead to a reduction in calories, but consuming a diet too low in carbohydrates is difficult to adhere to in the long- run. In addition, long-term, excessive high protein diets can cause liver and kidney damage. A study published in a 2012 edition of the "British Journal of Nutrition" reports that a reduced-calorie diet with a two-carbohydrate to one-protein ratio was most successful for diet adherence, body-fat reduction, and preservation of lean body mass. This agrees with the 50% carbohydrates, 25% protein, and 25% fat ratio noted above.

Fats are not necessarily bad for you, especially if you maintain a diet of good omega-3 healthy fats (olive, coconut, palm kernel). Dietary fat is a nutrient that helps your body absorb essential vitamins, maintains the structure and function of cell membranes, and helps keep your immune system working. Some types of fat, such as the omega-6 fats found in vegetable oils (safflower, corn, sunflower, peanut, soybean, and canola), may increase your risk of heart disease and other health problems. These fats also have more calories, increasing the risk of weight gain.

Another fact that most do not realize is that a continued diet that is high in calories will shorten one's lifespan. This is the result of the metabolic breakdown of food, which involves oxidation processes. The oxidation of food releases free radicals that cause inflammation in the body. Excessive inflammation from eating too many calories can shorten one's lifespan.

Healthy caloric intake for men and women depends on age and level of activity. Here is a basic guide showing calories per day intake ranges. The low end is for the more sedentary people, and the higher end is for the more active.

Children (age 2-3): 1000 to 1400 calories

Women (young): 1200 to 2200 calories
Women (middle age): 2000 to 2400 calories
Women (over 50): 1600 to 2200 calories

Men (young): 1800 to 2600 calories
Men (middle age): 2200 to 3000 calories
Men (over 50): 2000 to 2800 calories

From this guide, we see men need more calories than women do, and the middle-aged people require more than the younger or for those over 50 years old. Caloric intake exceeding these guidelines increases the number of free radicals, which cause inflammation, and shortens your life. Also, note that caloric restriction reduces the risk of heart arrhythmias and associated deaths.

The important aspect, then, is to consume just the right amount of nutrients so the body has balance without eating excessive calories. Is this possible? Can we eat food rich in nutrients and stay within the healthy total caloric intake? No . . . Not with our typical American diet! It consists of too much unhealthy fat and sugar. The most commonly eaten vegetable in the US is the potato—usually as a French fry or potato chip. The French fry is high glycemic sugar deep-fried in harmful omega-6 fats. The second most commonly eaten vegetable is the tomato, usually as ketchup, pasta sauce, or pizza sauce—loaded with sugar.

Sugar is an ingredient that makes us more addicted to food, causing people to overeat. It causes insulin spikes and the release of the ghrelin hormone, which makes us hungry and desire to eat more. Sugar is a quick fuel, but it also stimulates dopamine in the brain. Sugar can be more addictive than cocaine. You have undoubtedly seen some kids on a "sugar high". If you eat sweet foods, at least consume them *after* a meal so the sugar is absorbed more slowly into the blood stream and the insulin levels remain more even.

A great alternative to refined sugar is the natural plant based sweetener called Stevia. It is 150 times sweeter than sugar, stable at high heat (great for baked goods), and non-fermentable so cancer tumor cells are not able to metabolize it for energy. Also, remember a basic rule: if harmful and unhealthy foods are not in the kitchen, you will not be tempted to eat them. Shop for food in

CHAPTER TWO | THE HUMAN BODY

the supermarket on a full stomach, so impulsive junk foods will not end up in your shopping cart.

In order to live, our bodies need three components: air, water, and food. When our bodies need more air, we breathe harder, faster, and deeper. When we are in need of water, we feel thirsty and drink water until our brain says we have had enough. Yet, when we are hungry, how do we know we are eating nutritious food to feed and fuel the body? If we gorge ourselves, does that mean we have eaten what we need to sustain our body? The answer to this question is the key to maintaining a balance, and it reveals the second secret to develop a leaner, stronger body while avoiding cancer and other diseases.

The Second Secret is, efficiently obtain all the nutrients your body needs so that the ghrelin hormone turns off and the leptin hormone stays turned on. In this way, you will not feel hungry and crave to consume an excess of calories in the process (which, remember, also decreases lifespan). The key word here is "efficiently." When done right, you will not overeat, will not feel intense hunger pangs, and instead, will feel full of energy.

When I was growing up, I heard a strange story about a teenage girl who had an insatiable desire to eat dirt. Why would she do that? As it turned out, her body was iron deficient, and she ate dirt to absorb more iron into her body. The brain is very powerful and will do what it needs to survive. Her brain "instructed" her body to eat dirt in an attempt to get more iron. If you are eating many calories from food but are not getting the proper nutrients, the brain will tell the body to eat more food to try to get those nutrients via the ghrelin hormone. We can turn off this process so we do not overeat and pack around unwanted/unneeded pounds. *It is all about eating the right amount of food while obtaining all the required nutrients efficiently. That is, we should eat the right amount of the right kinds of foods.*

The purpose of food is for the body to obtain essential nutrients. If the body does not get them, the brain signals the ghrelin hormone to keep eating. This amounts to excessive calorie consumption, fat deposition, plus an unhealthy body.

The worst diet combination is omega-6 fats and simple processed sugar, especially high fructose corn syrup. Aside from overall weight gain, this also causes impairment of the learning and memory center in the brain—the hippocampus. The impairment can pass on to newborns when the pregnant mother eats this poor diet combination; and it is compounded even further when her offspring continues to consume the original poor diet. This process called **AGE's** (advanced glycation end products) occurs when sugar in the brain reacts with protein and causes the subsequent oxidation of the bad omega-6 fats, which damages the hippocampus. Likewise, as the acronym implies, it causes more rapid aging. AGE's can occur anywhere in the body where sugar, proteins, and omega-6 fats collide. Reverting to a healthy diet reverses the impairment, and reduces the inflammatory cytokines.

Frankly, the typical American diet doesn't provide enough essential nutrients in limited quantities to satisfy the needs of our body in a healthy manner. In addition, it is impossible to consume excessive calories and then to try to maintain that perfect body weight through rigorous exercise. Therefore, another method is necessary to accomplish this task. We will see later how supplementation with vitamins and nutrients will give the body all the vital resources to provide satiation and prevent the ghrelin hormone from causing unnecessary overeating while maintaining a healthy balance.

CHAPTER TWO | THE HUMAN BODY

Intermittent Fasting

THE PROCESS OF fasting has been around since ancient times and mentioned in the Bible: the Book of Luke: 18, verse 12 is one example—"I fast twice a week and give a tenth of all I get." Fasting is the abstinence of food and/or drink for a certain period. The individual can decide to fast one day each week, every other day, or even for several days.

Let us again look back to the time of the Garden of Eden. How did their lifestyle influence the way they nourished their body?

They lived simple lives without electricity, lights, or plumbing, and there definitely were no fast-food restaurants around the corner. There were no refrigerators to raid late at night and no fourth meals (really a "death meal" on steroids). Late night convenience stores were unheard of, no place to buy high glycemic chips deep-fried in rancid omega-6 oil, only to be washed down by soda pop containing HFCS (high fructose corn syrup) or artificial sweeteners. All they had was clean water and wholesome, fresh fruits and vegetables probably eaten during daylight hours.

This meant their window of opportunity to eat was around eight hours per day, every day; and this was after they went "gathering" to obtain their meal.

Lab mice studies have determined the impact of eating times on animal weight. Those mice with restricted eating times of eight hours each day were thin and in contrast, the mice that had unrestricted eating opportunity were obese.

The total caloric intake for both groups of mice was the same; the only difference was the timing of the meals. The interesting discovery was that the obese mice became thin too when they ate the restricted timeframe diet. Thus, intermittent fasting is **The Third Secret** to develop a leaner, stronger body while avoiding cancer and other diseases—eat during a set timeframe.

The intermittent fasting protocol that works best for humans is the eight-hour window during each day, every day. The period may differ for each individual due to work schedule, but the important factor is to maintain the eight-hour timeframe.

So what do you eat during the day? It is best to eat fresh vegetables, fruits, healthy fats, and protein, while restricting all refined sugar and high glycemic foods. Eat smaller meals but more frequently. Meals in which the total caloric content exceeds seven hundred calories will cause the body to place the extra calories into fat storage.

My personal timeframe is to eat between the hours of 11am and 7pm. The reason for this is due to my work and sleep pattern. It is best to stop eating three to four hours before bedtime. This helps prevent insomnia from eating foods that stimulate the brain and acid reflux which can later turn into esophageal cancer.

Here are some helpful facts to prevent acid reflux: avoid an alcohol nightcap, which relaxes the stomach sphincter and allows stomach acid to enter the esophagus; avoid soda pop, which is highly acidic; and limit milk chocolate and ice cream, which have a high fat content.

When starting out on an intermittent fasting protocol, it is best to ease into the pattern. Start by increasing the length of time between dinner and bedtime—until it is three to four hours. Then gradually increase the length of time between waking and eating the first meal. This can be done by adding one hour to each interval for a week and then increasing it by another hour a week later;

until you have reached the target of an eight-hour eating window.

So that you do not feel famished by the process, during the fasting hours drink as much clean water as possible. This will keep you hydrated and provide a sense of satiation. Documented reports show that when we feel hungry, it is more likely that the body is craving and needing water, not food. Moreover, rest assured the protocols discussed in later sections would curb any intense hunger pangs. In fact, many times I have to remind myself to eat because I am not hungry, even though it may be noon or one o'clock.

Why is intermittent fasting beneficial to the body and how will it help maintain a desirable weight? Intermittent fasting helps to maintain steady levels of insulin, with no peaks and valleys to send the hormones leptin and ghrelin into uncontrollable cyclic overdrive that causes periods of intense hunger. When a low carbohydrate diet without refined sugar follows the period of intermittent fasting, the cells of the body will reprogram to burn the available glucose first, and then burn fat. This consumes the stored fat in the visceral abdominal areas, which releases more adiponectin that further burns even more fat. In addition, the increased insulin sensitivity allows for greater glucose uptake in the cells for mitochondrial use, so you also feel more energetic.

The benefits of intermittent fasting are improved insulin sensitivity and thus prevention and reversal of type-2 diabetes, reduced LDL and total cholesterol, reduced inflammation from decreased blood glucose, reduced blood pressure, reduction of life threatening visceral fat storage, and consumption of fewer total calories which slows the aging process.

Processed Foods

WE WILL NOW look at manufactured processed foods that end up in our stores and restaurants. They can have many different added ingredients for flavoring, preservation, bulking up, thickening, and may include dyes intended to make foods more appealing. Many of these agents can have adverse effects in the human body. First, we need to understand the concept of excitotoxicity.

Excitotoxicity is the process whereby excessive amounts of a substance will excite a brain nerve cell essentially to its death. Brain cells have various receptors on the cell wall surface that activate when certain chemicals bind to that receptor. When the specific receptor over-activates, it stimulates the cell to take in toxic amounts of calcium inside the cell. This in turn activates large quantities of enzymes that damage the cell structure and its DNA—hence the term excitotoxicity. During normal biological function, normal amounts of calcium enter the cell to carry out normal cell functions; it is only through excessive stimulation by other chemicals that excitotoxicity occurs. There are many excitotoxins, which include glutamate (MSG), aspartame (artificial sweeteners), sulfites, nitrates/nitrites, mercury, aluminum, pesticides/herbicides/ fungicides, and industrial/household chemicals. Take special notice that these excitotoxins are synergistic, which means that if taken together, they are more damaging than the additive effects of each one individually. You could think of it this way: 1 + 1 + 1 = 5.

Excitotoxicity is a slow continual process that over time will kill many brain cells. Different excitotoxins will affect different areas in the brain. The result of these excitotoxins can be clearly

CHAPTER TWO | THE HUMAN BODY

seen in dementias like Alzheimer's, Parkinson's, and ALS (Amyotrophic Lateral Sclerosis—Lou Gehrig's disease), where the cause is excitotoxicity, but the affected location in the brain is different.

Let's focus on the neurotransmitter glutamate, which is responsible for 90 percent of the brain's nerve transmissions: it stimulates the brain into alertness. Glutamate is a neurotoxin, as listed above, but used for most of the brain's nerve impulses. So how does it not cause excitotoxicity?

Nerve cells have glutamate pumps that pull extra-cellular glutamate into the nerve cells and keep glutamate levels outside the cells at a minimum. If this biological protection mechanism were absent, the horrific death of our brain would result. The problem arises when outside sources, such as food and other chemicals, provide an overwhelming supply of toxins that overpower the protective nerve mechanism.

We will now look at the food additives that that are excitotoxins: MSG, artificial sweeteners, nitrates, nitrites, and sulfites. We must be aware of these and minimize their ingestion.

MSG stands for monosodium glutamate, referred to in this text as glutamate. It is the salt form of glutamic acid where sodium replaces the hydrogen atom of the hydroxyl group. This flavor enhancer stimulates the brain into feeling good and wanting to eat more MSG. We have all heard of the "Chinese Restaurant headache" that people suffer after eating food from eateries using MSG. In this process, MSG passes through the blood-brain barrier and over-stimulates the brain cells to create an excitotoxic condition and the headache.

MSG damages the brain and can cause, or is associated with,

many other problems like obesity, diabetes, heart attack, stroke, atherosclerosis, abnormal sexual development in babies (inhibits formation of brain neurons responsible for gender development), immune problems (auto immune disorders), cancer, Alzheimer's, Parkinson's, ALS, and seizures. These diseases all stem from inflammation, which MSG easily promotes.

Unfortunately, the damage, if done at an early age, can be life-long. If a pregnant mother eats many foods with MSG, the developing fetus will absorb it through the placenta, which will damage brain development in the fetus. If it affects the hypothalamus, the brain center that regulates weight, the leptin receptors are destroyed for life, leaving the hunger hormone, ghrelin, to go unimpeded. This will cause the child to become obese in early childhood and throughout life. Obesity potentiates if the child continues to eat MSG-laden foods. We have all noticed that more children are obese today than in past decades. This is due to more MSG added into the foods we eat. Food manufacturers calculate that if our brains are stimulated to eat more MSG foods, sales and profits are likely to increase.

MSG stimulates glutamate receptors in the pancreas, the organ that increases insulin production. This results in a greater uptake of sugar in muscle cells and results in hypoglycemia (low, insufficient levels of sugar), with all its associated problems. We have seen how hypoglycemia can cause irritability. Could excessive MSG consumption in our contemporary American culture be one (among many) of the possible sources of increased road rage incidents on our highways? Food for thought!

Low blood-glucose levels induce a craving for sugar, which, along with the effect of MSG on the hypothalamus makes the person always feel hungry. The increased insulin release from eating more sugar generates the storage of more fat. *This vicious cycle leads to metabolic syndrome conditions of obesity, diabetes, and heart disease.* The only way to end the cycle is eliminate MSG from the diet.

MSG naturally occurs in tomatoes, cheese, potatoes, mushrooms, and other vegetables and fruits. Foods that have high levels of glutamate include the following: anything listed as soy (or edamame), meat gravies, tomato paste, peanuts, mushrooms (especially Portobello), cheese (especially parmesan), dried or condensed cow's milk, processed meats (hot dogs, sausages, sliced meats), red meats, commercial soups, and snack chips. Cooking high-glutamate foods releases the glutamate that has become concentrated in beef broth and stocks.

Federal law allows any food or ingredient with less than 99 percent pure MSG, be labeled by any name the manufacturer wants. Therefore, they hide the MSG ingredient under various names. When you see the following items listed on the food label, assume it has glutamate in it, and put it back on the grocer's shelf:

Autolyzed yeast
Barley malt
Bouillon and broth
Carrageenan
Caseinate (Calcium or Sodium)
Citric acid
Condensed milk (powdered)
Enzymes
Gelatin
Hydrolyzed proteins
Isolated protein
Maltodextrin

Natural flavoring

Seasonings

Soy protein (isolates or concentrates)

Soy sauce

Spices

Stock

Textured protein

Vegetable protein

Whey protein (isolate)

Xanthan Gum

Yeast extract

The following two ingredients are not glutamates but are usually present with glutamate: Disodium Guanylate and Disodium Inosinate. If you read these on the label, put that food back, too.

Carrageenan is a food ingredient made from seaweed, used to thicken foods such as yogurt and ice cream. Along with its inclusion as an MSG contributor, it also causes inflammation of the colon and generates cancer—another reason to avoid it.

Here is one last thought as to why a healthy diet is crucial for children. A poor diet can promote ADHD (attention deficit hyperactive disorder). I knew a child whose teacher thought the student should be on Ritalin for ADHD. The parents instead changed the child's diet to remove all glutamate, the brain excitatory component in food. The symptoms of ADHD soon disappeared, and the child performed much better in school. More benefits from eating nutritious, healthy food!

Artificial sweeteners are synthetically manufactured chemicals that taste sweet and replace sugar in many foods. The most common artificial sweeteners are aspartame, sucralose, saccharin, and neotame. They are present under the premise that

CHAPTER TWO | THE HUMAN BODY

they contain fewer calories and will therefore aid in weight loss. The first claim is true, but the second is far from true and quite the opposite—you will not lose weight by eating foods with artificial sweeteners, but actually gain weight. How can this happen?

Aspartame causes increased insulin production, which increases leptin hormone resistance. This leads to further increases in the hunger hormone ghrelin that increases appetite and promotes fat storage. Thus, one has a craving for more sugary foods, is less satisfied from a meal, and actually feels hungrier. Have you ever wondered why you are hungry soon after eating diet foods?

It is a vicious cycle: aspartame increases insulin, which makes you hungrier, so you eat more, and get more visceral fat. You then become obese and produce more cytokines that cause insulin resistance so the body produces more insulin, and on and on and on. Sugar is the other excitotoxin that also increases insulin levels. To avoid this harsh cycle, avoid artificial sweeteners, sugar, and MSG.

During the metabolic breakdown of aspartame, it degrades into glutamate, formaldehyde, and methanol. *Glutamate* is an excitotoxin, which kills brain cells; *formaldehyde* is a tissue fixative chemical used to preserve cells for microscopic biopsy examination; and *methanol* is highly toxic and not fit for consumption—it is an antifreeze ingredient . . . Yummy! Clearly, none of these by-products is healthy for human consumption. Aspartame can cause brain tumors in infants and damage proper brain development, commonly leading to seizures, mental retardation, and abnormal behaviors. Parents, please do not let your children eat or drink "diet" anything, especially diet sodas.

Sulfites preserve fruits, vegetables, and wine by their antibacterial/antifungal properties. Most common is sulfur dioxide, which converts into sulfite, found in wine.

Other forms are sodium sulfite, sodium or potassium bisulfate, and sodium or potassium metabisulfite. Foods that are high in sulfite include wine (especially white); dried fruits; lemon juice concentrate; shredded coconut; and dehydrated potatoes (I knew it, those instant mashed potatoes we had as kids were bad for you—yuck!).

Other foods with somewhat high levels are jam/jelly, corn syrup, guacamole, pickles/olives, shellfish (shrimp, scallops, crab, and lobster), soy protein, processed cheese, and beer.

Sulfites are excitotoxins that can cause headaches. This is why some people can't drink white wine, which is high in sulfites. Long-term consumption of sulfites affects the brain and leads to neurodegenerative disorders like Alzheimer's and Parkinson's, along with depression, panic attacks, and anxiety.

Sulfites will cause chronic inflammation and are associated with those problems linked to inflammation; it also makes cancers grow faster. Sulfites can even cause hives, itching, difficulty breathing, asthma-like bronchiole spasms, and reactions like anaphylactic shock—which can be fatal.

Avoid wines, especially white wines that have more sulfites, and drink only those wines without sulfites or at least reduced amounts. Avoid foods that have added sulfites. Some people are severely affected by sulfites while others are not; but the reaction to sulfites can be non-detectable and still cause chronic inflammation.

Nitrates/nitrites are chemical agents generally used to prevent meat spoilage, provide taste, add color, and prevent botulism. Its use has decreased about 70 percent over the years, as more food manufacturers are using ascorbate, erythorbate, and/or vitamin E to prevent the conversion of nitrites into N-nitrosamine, a powerful carcinogen.

Some foods that are commercially grown and found to be high in nitrates are spinach, collard greens, broccoli, and tomatoes, among others. However, this depends on the amount of nitrate fertilizer used. Nitrites levels found in foods are usually lower than nitrates. Also, note that well water can contain high amounts of nitrates/nitrites due to farm fertilizers.

Processed meats still contain nitrites/nitrates as a preservative. In addition, many processed meats include broth, flavorings, and other MSG inherent additives. Stay away from processed meat and thereby reduce potential brain inflammation, as well as pancreatic or colon cancer.

Bacon also has the nitrate preservative. These processed meats can be soaked in heated water for ten minutes to dissolve away these preservative salts. Wash poultry before cooking to remove bleach used in the processing plant. One last note about meat is that you want to slow-cook it so the protein does not turn that char-black crispy texture as seen from grilling—this is a carcinogen known as heterocyclic amines.

Food dyes in many different foods make them look better and more appetizing; some are obvious and others not so much. Some, made from natural foods, are healthy, but more expensive to obtain the dye extracts. Artificial dyes are less expensive and made from petroleum products. Each color has a specific number to designate artificial dyes for identification. Each dye has its own inherent concern, it is best to assume they can be harmful, so avoid them if possible.

Artificial flavors, found everywhere, are comprised of various chemicals to create a certain taste. They are not natural flavors, which would be more expensive to include in the food. Unfortunately, in modern society we rely on chemistry to concoct a cocktail of chemicals to satisfy our palate. Some of these can be detrimental to our health. Diacetyl is a four-carbon molecule made up of two acetic acid (vinegar) molecules joined together. It has a unique butter taste so is used in microwave popcorn—the problem is that heating this chemical in the microwave can lead to toxins that contribute to Alzheimer's disease. Please pass the buttered microwave popcorn . . . Now where am I? ☹

Preservatives lengthen the shelf life of food. There are many, but as you can guess, they are not beneficial to your health. We have already looked at nitrates and nitrites; let's look at a few more preservatives that are best to avoid.

BHA and BHT (butylated hydroxyanisole and butylated hydrozytoluene) prevent oils from becoming rancid by preventing oxidation. BHT is phasing out, and replaced by BHA, but this doesn't mean it is safer for consumption. The risks for both include cancer.

TBHQ (tertiary-butyl hydroquinone) also prevents the oils and fats in food from oxidizing and turning rancid; and prevents them from changing color to make food more appealing. The FDA lists these preservatives as GRAS (generally recognized as safe) but only in concentrations less than a certain amount. What happens if you eat many foods with this preservative in them? Reports state that five grams of TBHQ can kill you—this is not what I consider generally recognized as safe. It implies you know the exact amount in each food and the total amount of each food consumed so you can calculate the total number of grams. Maybe *you* can do this, but I think about other things when I eat.

Notice that food manufacturers will use many acronyms (BHA, BHT, and TBHQ). This makes the foods sound safer to eat, even though they are not. If they spell out a long, hard-to-pronounce name that sounds scary, the consumer may not buy it. The good news is that all these acronyms and long names can be deciphered on the internet. You are encouraged to research all ingredients for their safety, and with smart phones, it is even easier.

Sodium benzoate is the salt of benzoic acid and found in soda pop, salad dressing, and other foods. When combined with vitamin C, heat, and a long shelf life, the breakdown product is benzene—a known carcinogen. It has been associated with hyperactivity in children.

Azodicarbonamide is flour bleaching agent and dough conditioner in baked goods, but also found in yoga mats and shoe rubber. Yum!!! It can cause allergies, asthma, and cancer.

These are only a few of the food preservatives. There are also preservatives found in sunscreen, make-up, deodorant, and shampoo. Generally, the hazardous material found in sundries is parabens (parahydroxybenzoates), which are from benzene derivatives. Generally, anything made with benzene or a derivative is often a carcinogen.

Alum is another preservative found in pickle juice to maintain the crispy texture of pickles. The chemical composition is a sulfate salt that contains aluminum. It is also in baking powder to make bread whiter. As a known excitotoxin, avoid this ingredient. Some other forms of alum are found in flame-retardants, vaccines, and taxidermy to preserve the animal hide.

Inflammation

INFLAMMATION TRIGGERS THE biological response of the body to fight an invading organism, repair damaged cells and tissues, and/or rid harmful chemical irritants. It is a protective measure that involves cell-signaling mediator proteins (cytokines) to call the body into protective action. They induce blood vessels to transport reparative chemical agents and immune cells (white blood cells) to fight the inflammation. Its purpose is to stop the cause of tissue injury, remove damaged cells, and start the tissue repair process. This is short-term inflammation, which alleviates a crisis without causing damage to the surrounding cells or tissues.

The real problem occurs when the insult to the body remains over a long period. Often the persistent inflammation leads to unwanted damage of the adjacent healthy tissues—collateral damage. Thus, **chronic inflammation** (long-term inflammation) is very destructive and leads to most diseases and ailments.

As a result, chronic inflammation causes diseases to appear sooner, more frequently, and more severely. Some examples of these diseases are diabetes, autoimmune disorders, periodontitis (gum disease), cancer, arthritis, atherosclerosis, heart disease, and stroke. Chronic inflammatory brain diseases include ALS, Parkinson's, and Alzheimer's.

There are various causes of inflammation. Free radicals generated via metabolism in mitochondria are one source; this is why it is best to limit total caloric consumption to only what the body needs for proper biological function. Excessive calories create an excess of free radicals. Bacteria and viruses cause inflammation. Visceral fat generates inflammatory cytokines from its presence, so it is prudent to decrease belly fat as much as possible. AGE's are another source of inflammation: in this case, excess blood sugar reacts with protein to create the oxidation of fat.

Free radicals will cause lipid peroxidation of cell walls, which are predominantly lipids. When the cell wall oxidizes, it creates wall damage and loss of structural integrity, leaving cellular contents unprotected. This creates inflammation.

The brain can acquire inflammation as well. In fact, the brain can be inflamed while the body is not; but if the body is inflamed, so too is the brain. Excitotoxic agents will cause brain inflammation: glutamate (MSG), aspartame (artificial sweeteners), sulfites, nitrates/nitrites, mercury, aluminum, pesticides/herbicides/fungicides, and industrial/household chemicals.

Sugar is another brain excitotoxin. It stimulates the dopamine receptors, and the free radicals from metabolism cause oxidation of fat (AGE's). Remember, the brain is 60 percent fat!

The brain is 5 percent of body weight but consumes 25 percent of the glucose and 20 percent of the oxygen required for metabolism, which creates an abundance of free radicals.

Aging and a decrease in production of the mitochondria deprive the brain of energy and magnifies the effects of excitotoxicity and inflammation. Luckily, for humanity, the brain has a separate immune system to deal with inflammation—the microglia (discussed shortly).

Oxidation/Reduction

WHAT DOES IT mean when oxidation occurs? **Oxidation** of a molecule is the structural loss of electrons (a gain in positive overall charge) while **reduction** is marked by a gain in electrons (a gain in negative overall charge). It could involve one or more electrons, depending on each component. This process explains how free radicals oxidize a molecule by transferring electrons to that recipient molecule, which then becomes reduced by the addition of the electrons. Oxidation usually involves the oxygen atom of the molecule, as it can readily donate electrons. Think of oxygen as an oxidizer that gives up electrons.

The addition of electrons changes the physical nature of the recipient molecule, and in the human body, causes harmful effects if not reversed.

Antioxidants prevent molecular/cellular destruction—they are the sacrificial agents that take the electron(s) from the free radical so it cannot oxidize other biologically important molecules and cause damage. Free radicals can otherwise cause chain reactions in cells, leaving damage and cell death in the process. The antioxidants stop this from happening.

Oxidation is crucial for life, as metabolism in the mitochondria via the citric acid cycle produces necessary ATP energy but also creates harmful free radicals. This is why a low total caloric diet that supplies just enough energy is beneficial for a healthy body while reducing the creation of excessive free radicals and thus oxidative stress on the body. If there is less oxidative stress and reduced inflammation, there is less cell damage and death.

The human body utilizes many antioxidants to prevent chronic inflammation. Five main antioxidants are part of the antioxidant network.

The Antioxidant Network

THE NETWORK INCLUDES vitamin C, vitamin E, lipoic acid, ubiquinol (a form of CoQ10), and glutathione. These five main antioxidants protect cells from free radical and lipid peroxidation damage by accepting excess electrons. The minerals magnesium, selenium, and zinc aid their antioxidant properties.

The location in the cell where the antioxidant is most effective depends primarily on its solubility. Fat-soluble antioxidants will benefit the cell phospholipid wall, and the water-soluble ones will benefit the cytosol portion of the cell. Note that some are co-soluble and affect both water and fat-soluble cell components.

Vitamin C and vitamin E complement each other due to their differing solubility. Vitamin C is water-soluble and is most effective in the cytosol. Vitamin E is fat-soluble and is most effective in the cell membranes. So between the two, they are cross protective in both phases of cell solubility.

CoQ10 has three reduction states: fully oxidized (ubiquinone), partially oxidized (semiquinone), and the fully reduced form—ubiquinol. Because ubiquinol is the fully reduced form, it is the better supplement to obtain. Ubiquinol is co-soluble and is effective in both the cell membrane and the cytosol.

Glutathione is effective in both the nucleus, which protects the DNA, and in the cytosol. It is very important in liver detoxification. Glutathione is synthesized from three amino acids: glutamic acid, glycine, and cysteine. Since cysteine is the limiting factor for its synthesis, supplementation with N-acetyl-cysteine (NAC) promotes the formation of glutathione.

Lipoic acid is the universal antioxidant as it functions in all three cellular compartments—the nucleus, the cytosol, and the cell membrane—and will remain a potent antioxidant even after receiving donated electrons.

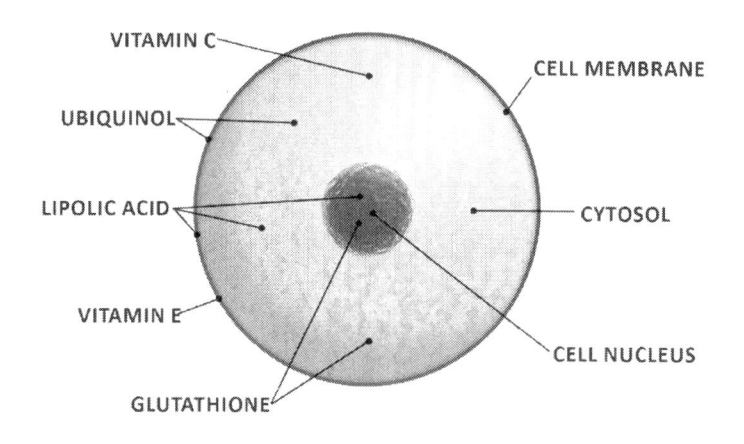

NETWORK ANTIOXIDANTS
AND THEIR TARGETS TO REDUCE
INFLAMMATION IN HUMAN CELLS

All five antioxidants work synergistically well together and it is best to supplement them as a group. They help each other to get back into their reduced state so they can be powerful antioxidants once again.

The Immune System

THE IMMUNE SYSTEM relies on two components to fight infection and inflammation: *humoral and cellular immunity*. Humoral immunity, or **antibody-mediated immunity**, involves large molecules of antibodies found in the humors, or body fluid spaces. When the body detects a foreign invader that has a special cell wall marker (**antigen**), it attaches an antibody to it—like two puzzle pieces fitting together. There are thousands of antigens and their corresponding antibodies. Antibodies are specific for, and only bind to one particular antigen. The body will recognize this invader as foreign and send the cell-mediated immune cells to destroy it. Thus, antibodies support immunity by attaching to antigens of invading organisms, marking them for destruction by the cellular immune components.

Cellular immunity involves of the release of cytokines in response to the detected antigens along with the attraction of white blood cells to confront foreign material in the body. These white blood cells consist of macrophages, neutrophils, monocytes, mast cells, lymphocytes and eosinophils—these do the most work in killing and breaking down invading organisms. Macrophages not only engulf and destroy bacteria, viruses and fungi, but they will also gobble up (**phagocytosis**) any inflammatory cellular debris, cancer cells, and foreign material, then rid the body of it.

Often the damage from the immune system, in response to inflammation, is more severe than the invading organism itself. Normal inflammatory responses rid the body of unwanted materials and the tissues heal without incident. However, chronic inflammation leads to prolonged immune responses that present an adverse situation. This is when the surrounding normal tissues suffer the intense attack from immune cells and the free radicals released to kill off invaders. This long-term assault leads to chronic inflammation and more cellular immune response, which leads to more inflammation and more cellular immune response, and on and on and on. *This is why diseases and cancer occurs. You can see why it is important to limit inflammation so the immune response will not lead to other ailments.*

Eighty percent of immune activity occurs in the intestines and colon, promoted by probiotics or the good bacteria; this is the point of entry for organisms and toxins that come from food. Cells lining the GI tract and respiratory tract secrete the IgA (immunoglobulin A) antibody, which binds to these organisms and toxins to prevent entry into the blood. It is important to eat a healthy diet, promote gut health with probiotics and other supplements, and exercise so the immune system can function well.

Aging is associated with decreased immune function, which can lead to chronic inflammation, and cytokine release that can eventually lead to cancer. People who smoke also have a disadvantage in that immune cells have nicotine receptors. Smoking chronically suppresses cellular immunity and causes more infections, colds, sinusitis, bladder infections, and the flu.

There is a direct link between gut health, body health, and brain health. This in turn is associated with gum disease due to the presence of oral inflammatory bacteria. The body is a clearly a highly inter-connected system and operates as such. It all boils down to inflammation and the immune system's reaction in the body to counteract the cause.

Microglia

THE BRAIN HAS nerve cells consisting of axons and dendrites. The axons are long threadlike parts of a nerve cell along which impulses conduct from the nerve cell body to other nerves.

Dendrites are the small projections from the nerve cell body that receive impulses from other nerve cells. The nerve connections or synapses allow impulses to relay transmitted signals from one nerve cell to another. They transmit electrical impulses, using glutamate as the main neurotransmitter. There are also nonneural or glial cells that provide support and protection for the nerves. A type of glial cell is part of the brain's own immune system, called the **microglia**. They are macrophage cells that function similar to that of the body's cellular immune system, but are confined to the brain and spinal cord and separated by the blood-brain barrier.

The microglial cell will scavenge for infection, damaged nerve cells, and **beta-amyloid plaque**. A build-up of beta-amyloid plaque, or excessive protein in patients with dementia, is due to aging and diminished microglial capability to fight inflammation.

When foreign material does enter the brain, the microglia act quickly to phagocytize it and decrease the inflammation before nerve damage occurs. This is critical since there is no humoral immunity in the brain and because the antibodies are too large to cross the blood-brain barrier.

Most damage in the brain is by chronic microglial activation, due to excitotoxicity in response to extra-cellular glutamate from the body's poor diet—for example, eating too much soy for a long time. Microglial cytokines cause glutamate receptors to be hypersensitive and magnify excitotoxicity. When this process occurs for a long time, it overpowers the ability of the microglia to remove the beta-amyloid plaque, and brain damage is results.

Artificial sweeteners can also cause excitotoxicity and over stimulation of the microglia. Many other agents can over-activate microglia cells like pesticides, viruses, bacteria, stress, and vaccine adjuvants such as mercury and aluminum. Brain injury and trauma can initiate the brain's microglial immune system as well.

Aging causes chronic inflammation, and along with higher glutamate levels in the elderly, this will cause chronic activation of the microglia and thus more excitotoxicity, which leads to neurodegenerative diseases such as Parkinson's and Alzheimer's. This is a critical matter; today we see this issue in the higher occurrence of dementia in our older family members

Vaccines

VACCINES FUNCTION ONLY by promoting the antibody-mediated immune process, stimulating the production of specific antibodies for the organism in the inoculation. For antibodies to be effective, the invading organism (**pathogen**) must have an antigen for which the host body has the complementary antibody. If the vaccine-induced antibodies do not correctly match the antigen from, say, a flu bug that infects the world that year, the vaccine-induced antibodies are ineffective, and will not increase immunity or protect people. This is why it is important for vaccine manufacturers to know specifically which strain of flu they intend to guard against.

Another failing of vaccines is that antibody production may provide the host some protection for a limited time. However, after a while, if the invading organism mutates, that will require a new antibody to combat the mutated invader. This is why vaccine companies advised "boosters," to stimulate the body to produce updated antibodies. Nevertheless, they too, have limited effects.

Acquired immunity, on the other hand, developed within the body from the actual disease, provides life-long cellular immunity. Here, the sensitized T lymphocytes are primed from the pathogen, so that whenever that pathogen is encountered again—even decades later—the cell-mediated response will destroy it. *This results in lifetime immunity.*

Cellular immunity is, therefore, what needs fortification instead of immunity through artificially means (vaccines). Cellular immunity is the workhorse of the immune system and is most beneficial in protecting the body from harmful diseases.

As a child, my mother made sure all of her children were exposed to measles, mumps, chicken pox, and German measles when one of us got the disease. As a result, we developed life-long cellular immunity for these diseases and a stronger immune system in general. With modern medicine today, any potential harmful effects from these diseases can be mitigated, so much so that the benefit of natural immunity still outweighs the risks of limited vaccine immunity and vaccines' harmful additives. The only painful aspect from the mumps that I experienced was when my brother accidently hit me in the neck—ouch! I survived the accidental assault and now have lifetime immunity toward the mumps.

The concept of **herd immunity**, heralded by the pro-vaccination camp, is not the ultimate reason to vaccinate our society against diseases. They claim this is the only way to protect yourself and children from disease. However, let us look at herd immunity and see why it is ineffective in our social environment.

Herd immunity utilizes the principle that if most people are currently immune to a disease, then they (the herd) protect the susceptible non-immune minority, since the probability of spreading the pathogen to them is low. If there is very little pathogen floating around because most people's bodies destroy it, then the chance of passing it on to others is remote.

For herd immunity to be effective, 90 to 100 percent of the population must be immune to a disease. Is herd immunity attainable? Immunity through vaccination is antibody-mediated immunity that lasts on average two to four years and then tapers off. Flu vaccines produce protective antibodies in 30 to 60 percent of people because flu vaccine manufacturers guess at which strain to protect against—and they often get it wrong, as seen in America during the winter of 2014/15. Thus, herd immunity for the flu can never occur because the level of immunity for the herd never attains the required level.

Dr. J. Anthony Morris, former chief vaccine control officer and research virologist for the FDA stated, "There is no evidence any influenza vaccine is effective . . . The producers of these vaccines know they are useless, but go on selling them."

He also stated, "There is a great deal of evidence to prove that immunization of children does more harm than good. "

We have seen that vaccines have limited effectiveness. Another example of this was the outbreak of measles at Disneyland, California, in early 2015. Many of those who contracted the measles already had measles vaccinations, and of the 147 people who got sick at the park, there were no reported deaths.

An interesting statistic is that there were only 440 reported deaths from measles during the period of recorded history *before* the vaccine was ever developed. The risks and deaths from measles vaccines far outnumber deaths from the disease itself.

Panic was rampant from the Disneyland outbreak as the parents of vaccinated children did not want their own children exposed to the non-vaccinated ones. However, logic dictates that with a vaccinated child you would not have to worry. If you believe vaccines protect you against that disease, then you have nothing to fear—unless there is really no sure vaccine protection against the measles in the first place. Since there were no deaths from the measles outbreak at Disneyland, is it really worth taking the risks to vaccinate?

People take great risks in vaccination, but the pharmaceutical companies, some healthcare professionals, and the media cover it up—putting profit before ethics. Remember, vaccines are a multi-billion dollar industry. Also, keep in mind that many vaccines contain various adjuvants that cause harmful side effects. Thimerosal, Aluminum, formaldehyde, and MSG, are some of the detrimental additives listed on the CDC website for each vaccine. See Appendix A for a list of Vaccines and their added adjuvants. Let's look at these harmful adjuvants in more detail.

Thimerosal is a preservative comprised of 50% mercury, which inhibits enzymes that would neutralize free radicals and blocks the removal of glutamate from the nervous system. Thus, it stimulates the immune system and encourages an inflammatory reaction, which it does very well. Mercury accumulates in microglia cells and promotes excitotoxins and glutamate production, which degenerate the brain, ultimately causing dementia. For these reasons, I stopped placing mercury fillings in my patients' teeth, years ago, even though the ADA still deems mercury fillings "safe." It's true that mercury is chelated (bound) to other elements in the alloy, but it still manages to leach out during chewing and the grinding of teeth. As a dentist, I refuse to take chances with my patients' health.

Aluminum interferes with and inhibits over 200 needed biological functions. It causes brain excitotoxicity by activating the microglia immune system. The microglia secretes the inflammatory cytokine TNF-alpha (tumor necrosis factor-alpha), which causes brain inflammation and leads to dementia. *The good* *news is that the mineral magnesium inhibits the effects of glutamate,* probably by forming the salt called magnesium glutamate, which does not allow it to bind to the microglial receptors, and thus inhibits stimulation of the inflammatory immune TNF-alpha cytokine.

Aluminum also inhibits the mitochondrial citric acid cycle ATP energy production, thus giving the brain less energy and increases sensitivity to excitotoxicity. Why is this so important? It is because the brain is extremely energy dependent. Without energy, brain cells die leading to the many brain diseases we see today.

For people with kidney disease and/or failure, it is very important to refrain from vaccines with aluminum as the kidneys cannot excrete the aluminum, so it builds up and can cause total kidney failure. Patients would then require expensive, time-consuming dialysis treatment.

As with the production of the salt magnesium glutamate mentioned above, aluminum forms the salt called aluminum glutamate, which readily absorbs from the GI tract and crosses the blood-brain barrier. The glutamate can then activate microglia receptors that stimulate the immune response to increase inflammation in the brain. Aluminum can also concentrate in the myelin sheath of neural pathways (the protective layer around nerves) and cause the degenerative autoimmune disease multiple sclerosis.

Here is a key reminder: *The effects of mercury and aluminum are cumulative in the brain and over time continue their damage. Unless one takes specific nutrients to bind and remove these poisons, they are there for life.*

Formaldehyde is another harmful additive to vaccines. Mortuaries preserve our loved-ones by using embalming fluid, which contains formaldehyde. I don't know about you, but I only want to be embalmed once—and not before I'm dead! That's not to say that there is enough formaldehyde in a vaccine to embalm an entire body. Rather, there is enough poison to kill healthy cells around the injection site. This can lead potentially to chronic inflammation and a cytokine release, which leads to other serious outcomes such as cancer. Have you ever noticed the intense red, swollen, hot tissue around a vaccination site? Inflammatory cytokines are doing their damage.

As if not all of this was bad enough, the vaccine schedule commonly recommended for everyone—from newborns to developmental maturity is alarming in its excessiveness. It is "recommended" that kids have 26 vaccines by their first birthday, 40 by the time they reach school age, and 150 during a person's lifetime. This level of vaccination intake allows for the accumulation in the brain of an excess of neurotoxins, providing the chemical and physiological foundation for even greater chances of dementia and Alzheimer disease at earlier stages in life. Yet, it's precisely because vaccinations are so lucrative that vaccine companies bombard the FDA continually for approval of more and more new vaccines. When will this vaccine insanity end?

Natural infections incurred over a lifetime induce lifelong immunity without the need for "boosters." Indeed, naturally acquired immunity to the flu can give protection for years down the road, even when the flu mutates into a virus similar in form to what it was in years or decades past. What is important to understand is that this cannot happen with flu vaccines.

Multiple vaccines such as DPT (diphtheria, pertussis, tetanus) increase the risk of autoimmune diseases such as asthma and juvenile diabetes. In addition, some claim that it can also lead to autism—as explored below.

Live virus vaccines (measles/mumps/rubella, smallpox, and chickenpox) should be avoided, because even though they attenuate, or weaken, the viral wall fragments can imbed in organs only to create hidden allergies, which can then cause chronic inflammation and even cancer down the line. Due to free radical immune responses, these viral particles can mutate into another virus and cause unrelated diseases, such as multiple sclerosis, or cause immune suppression leading to the development of a secondary infection, such as pneumonia.

Autism, too, has been linked to vaccines. In 1975, autistic children were one in 5,000. This baseline value resulted from natural genetic disposition. In 1990, the autism rate exploded to one in 500 or a ten-fold increase, which some researchers argue correlates to the prevalent and widespread use of vaccines. This phenomenon is disturbing because of its implications beyond just this country. Expansion of worldwide vaccination programs caused a global pandemic. Infants' brain development is most fragile in the first two years of life, yet the brain continues to mature until around age 25. Vaccines containing thimerosal and the adjuvant aluminum correlate with increased numbers of autism. Mercury and aluminum are synergistic and cause neural degenerative autistic defects in children's brains.

The genetic link would account for the fact that not all children developed autism from the vaccines, as seen with the baseline rate in 1975; but the genetic rate is constant and would not increase. Therefore, the only way to account for the dramatic rise in autism, including globally, is from vaccines. With the autism rate jumping to one in every 68 children, that is close to a 700 percent increase! There is simply no stronger evidence and explanation for this horrific problem other than the extreme increase in the number of vaccines inflicted on our precious youth. Please review the chart below.

Autism Rates in America

1975: 1 in 5,000

1985: 1 in 2,500

1995: 1 in 500

2000: 1 in 150

2004: 1 in 125

2006: 1 in 110

2008: 1 in 88

2010-2014: 1 in 68

Sources: cdc.gov, autismspeaks.org

Over-activation of the microglia is a process that starts from priming the microglia. This event initiates the immune system to produce an intense **cytokine storm** to generate a strong inflammatory reaction upon subsequent inoculation thereby releasing a large quantity of cytokines (or storm). It is comparable to cases of poison oak exposure, in which the victim may not react upon first exposure but upon further exposure experiences a full-blown and relentless itchy rash.

Vaccinations produce higher levels of immune activation and

the immune response can persist longer than with natural infections—sometimes lasting years. When the elderly already have primed microglia and repeated frequent vaccinations, the result could worsen any preexisting neurological disorder or even initiate such a disorder. Thus, the risk of Alzheimer's disease and Parkinson's magnifies.

Mercury is fat-soluble (the brain is 60 percent fat), so it will accumulate in the brain. Some vaccines have phased out thimerosal, but flu vaccines still contain mercury. For people over 55, if you have five years of continuous flu vaccinations, this increases chances of Alzheimer's by 1000 percent. This fact alone makes the extreme risk not worth the benefit and the reason why I refuse vaccinations for the flu.

In the fetus, the priming of microglia may come from vaccinating the mother during pregnancy from a "recommended" flu vaccine. In this case, the toxins pass through the placenta to the fetus. Alternatively, it may occur with the first vaccine inoculation, usually at birth with the hepatitis B vaccine.

Once the microglia is primed, subsequent vaccinations will trigger a full microglial activation. Excessive frequency for vaccinations, especially within months of a previous inoculation, can magnify the affects. The resulting cytokine storm in the developing brain can result in abnormal development, potentially leading to autism and/or obesity in early life and dementia in later life.

After talking to a first-time mom who was tending to her crying two-month-old, she gave her child a liquid in a plastic tube. Curiosity compelled me to ask what it was. She said her newborn just received four "routine" vaccines at the pediatrician's office and had a rash and fever, for which she gave children's Tylenol.

CHAPTER TWO | THE HUMAN BODY

Not wanting to alarm her, I did not tell her that the vaccines are causing an inflammatory cytokine storm that is resulting in the fever and rash that was causing the baby to cry incessantly. Moreover, to add insult to injury—quite literally—she just gave the child the pediatrician-prescribed acetaminophen, which is a known agent that can cause irreparable liver damage and further hinders the child's detoxification process by inhibiting the antioxidant glutathione. Thus, there is an increased chance the child will suffer autism early in development, liver damage, and possibly even death.

Then I asked if she signed a consent form for her baby to receive the vaccinations, to which she replied, "No." The physician's staff informed her it was the routine vaccination schedule, and proceeded with the injections.

To perform any type of procedure on a patient, the healthcare provider needs to obtain consent from the patient or guardian. This is not a haphazard implication, but a well-defined process. It does not necessarily have to be signed consent, but the pediatrician would be wise to make it a signed consent process for vaccinations. For true consent to happen, there are four steps. These steps are:

1) a description of the Procedure

2) noting any Alternatives to the procedure

3) noting any Risk associated with the procedure

4) asking if there are any Questions.

The acronym for this process is **PARQ**, pronounced as park, or pronounced by enunciating each letter. For vaccinations, the "procedure" would sound something like this: "The vaccine is injected into the thigh (or shoulder), there may be a rash and swelling that could last 3 to 5 days, and the baby may be irritable and cry during this time." The "alternative," of course, is to decline the vaccination.

Then, all of the possible "risks" should be discussed. From what you have read above, do you think many parents receive this information about all the possible risks? This step must also include the possibility of death . . . Unfortunately deaths have occurred and been documented.

This is probably something few parents are told, because a prudent parent may look into the matter more closely and decline the vaccine. I hope you now feel well informed as to the risks; whether you choose to give consent is up to you.

The last step is to answer any "questions" that you as a concerned parent may have. Questions you should ask may be something like the following:

"What is the morbidity (how often harm occurs) and mortality (the chance of death) risk of the vaccine?"

"Did you as a pediatrician give ALL these vaccines on schedule to your own children? If not, why not?"

"Will you be accountable for any adverse reaction?"

This is the proper medical procedure for obtaining consent. I doubt many parents have witnessed this process. I thank God that my children received far fewer vaccines than the recommended ones today; and if I had it to do over again, they would not have gotten as many as they did. I would research all aspects of the proposed vaccines and make informed decisions. This is our duty as their parents, to protect and nurture them throughout childhood so they can live to become healthy, happy, dynamic adults.

Many vaccines are marginally efficacious, as the effect of preventing the disease is non-existent, short-lived, or incomplete.

Nutrition, sanitation, and supplements to improve the immune system have done more to prevent disease than vaccines. Also, remember that increased mercury and aluminum can increase risk for Alzheimer's disease later in life.

Studies also show you have a good chance of developing Guillian-Barre Syndrome from receiving the flu vaccination. To remind you of what we covered above, the flu vaccine causes an intense immune reaction resulting in a cytokine storm. This is an autoimmune disorder, similar to multiple sclerosis, where the nerves become dysfunctional and causes muscle weakness and pain. It can even be fatal. Much more research is required to produce safe and effective vaccines—I just do not want to be the guinea pig for the research! In a personal aside, sadly, my own father developed Guillian-Barre Syndrome after just one flu vaccination. The precautionary measures I encourage you to undertake derive from my own real-life experiences.

GMO Foods

EVOLUTION PROVIDED NATURAL selection or breeding, of plants and animals. The genetic traits are blended together to form a composite life form. There was no intervention from humans, and the process was very random. Then along came selective breeding, around 12,000 BC, when humans crossbred plants and animals with desirable genetic traits to create characteristics that are more beneficial. This process did not involve the manipulation of the genetic code or the genetic sequence of the organism.

In 1973, genetic engineering led to the development of **GMOs** (genetically modified organisms). In this process, the genetic material of an organism becomes altered by the mutation, insertion, or deletion of genes through biotechnology. Companies such as Monsanto, DuPont, Bayer, Syngenta, and Dow commercialized this technology in 1976. They produce and sell GMO seeds, GMO food, and GMO medicine. For our purposes we will focus on GMO seeds and food; you are encouraged to research GMO medicines.

The focus for developing GMO seeds and the plants that grow from them, was to insert specific genetic material into the plant gene sequence to provide specific desired traits.

The hope was to increase crop yield even in drought areas, make the plant resistant to bugs and weed killer, and make the food more nutritious.

Monsanto is a chemical company that manufactures Roundup® (with the weed killer ingredient called glyphosate). They wanted to develop a seed that would produce a plant that would not die from the use of Roundup. They inserted genes into the seeds that produced characteristics in the plant to make it resilient to the weed killer. In effect, the farmer could use Roundup® on their crops to kill obnoxious weeds while saving the intended crop. This technology led to the implantation of genes to have the plant produce its own insecticide; thus, if an insect ate the plant leaf, the insect would soon die. Isn't this great? Monsanto had created plants that were both weed killer-tolerant and contain their own inherent bug killer. But wait—it gets worse!

Since the development of these GMO seeds, farmers discovered that the first year of these crops provided good yields, and the weeds and insects were not a problem. Then came the following years when the weeds developed a resistance to glyphosate. Today, they have reached the point where much more glyphosate must be applied to control weeds; and the super weeds that developed require other, more hazardous chemicals for control.

A Washington State University study concluded that ten times more glyphosate is now necessary to control the weed problem. The millions of pounds of glyphosate used are polluting the air, rivers, and lakes, and are contaminating the soil. It is even finding its way into well water that people drink. People tested for glyphosate residues are showing high concentrations of this poison. An article by Mike Barrett, dated May 4, 2014, discusses this fact (see http://naturalsociety.com/3-studies-proving-toxic-glyphosate-found-urine-blood-even-breast-milk/). In addition, the butterfly and bee populations have been decimated from glyphosate, leaving beekeepers struggling to keep healthy, active hives while leaving the rest of the world wondering about the dire consequences to the ecosystem of drastic drops in both populations.

In order to assure safety for human consumption, the FDA requires testing of GMO foods before placement on store shelves. Monsanto performed the testing, and, not surprisingly, they found these GMO foods to be safe. Talk about the wolf guarding the hen house! Let's take a look at the study performed by Monsanto.

The experiment involved lab rats fed biotech corn containing intrinsic glyphosate residue. The rat study lasted for *ninety days*, or the equivalent age of early adulthood in humans. Their research team found no health hazards from their study. So far, so good, right? Now let us look at an independent study conducted by a neutral-party outside research group.

A study by Gilles-Eric Seralini at the University of Cain in France and the Department of Neurological Sciences at the University of Verona, Italy, performed an analysis on the safety of

GMO corn and residues of the pesticide Roundup®. They published their results in the journal "Food and Chemical Toxicology." Their study lasted *two years*, which is the entire lifespan of the lab rat and corresponds to a *full lifespan in humans*. This study determined that glyphosate causes breast cancer in female rats and liver/kidney cancer in male rats. The only difference between the Monsanto and Seralini studies was the length of calendar time the rats were observed for tumor development—90 days versus two years. The conclusion is that given appropriate time, cancer will develop from GMO foods, even though it may be in later years of human life. If you want to see horrifying pictures of the lab rats with massive tumors, look up the study on the internet. Monsanto prefers you do not research these facts, and instead blindly consume their GMO foods.

There have been statewide initiatives to pass labeling laws. Vermont passed one such labeling law that went into effect in 2016; Monsanto has sued the state of Vermont over this labeling issue but lost in the Supreme Court. One would think that if a company was proud of their innovative research and that if GMOs were so safe, they would want everyone to know this and would label it accordingly . . . Unless Monsanto has something to hide.

The Right-to-Know label initiatives failed in California, Washington, and Oregon (by only 800 votes) directly due to the millions of dollars spent by negative and misleading advertising by the corporations themselves—who want to keep people in the dark. This is why Monsanto and others are lobbying the U.S. Congress to pass the bill that is popularly dubbed "the Dark Act"—Deny Americans the Right-to-Know Act. If passed, it would deny every state in the country the ability to pass GMO labeling laws. The good news is that the bill failed to pass the senate in March 2016, but it was very close.

In 2015, the International Agency for Research on Cancer (IARC), the specialized cancer agency of the World Health Organization, has assessed the carcinogenicity of the herbicide glyphosate and classified it as *probably carcinogenic* to humans. Another alarming fact about genetically modified food is that genetically altered food consumed by humans can have the GMO-altered-DNA enter human cells and embed in human DNA—which can then pass on through three human generations. No telling what mutations could occur.

One final problem to note is that GMO crops can cross-pollinate with natural plants and forever alter their genetic makeup—and we would have no recourse. Mankind must insure that heirloom seeds, free of GMOs, always survive to maintain unadulterated foods. With all this information coming forth about GMOs, it would be prudent to avoid all foods that contain GMOs; and that means becoming an avid food label reader.

Read Food Labels

IN TODAY'S WORLD, it is imperative that we read and accurately interpret food labels. The health and well-being of our families depend on this. As seen above, labels can be misleading, and the FDA does not help by allowing misinformation to continue. Remember, if you cannot pronounce the ingredient, or if acronyms designate the ingredient, it probably is not healthy. Look up names of ingredients to make sure they are safe to eat. Let's run through a few examples of actual labels to determine if the ingredients are safe.

The first example is seasoning salt. There are many flavor enhancers on store shelves, and I randomly picked one up to read the label. On the yellow label it has the red-circle, backslash symbol (the no symbol ⊘) with the acronym "MSG" in bold, black print. We would think that this product has no MSG within the seasoning salt. For added assurance, the manufacturer placed the words "contains no added monosodium glutamate" around the red circle. So we should feel safe this product has no MSG, right. Don't be too hasty! Read the back label for ingredients.

The ingredients listed on the container are in the following order: Salt, sugar, paprika, pepper, garlic, soy sauce powder (soybeans, wheat, salt, and maltodextrin), cellulose gel & citric acid. It contains soy & wheat.

Two things should jump right out to tell us this product has MSG in the salt. What are they?

From the list of known ingredients to have MSG, we see soy sauce and maltodextrin. This product definitely has MSG, due to the inclusion of soy and maltodextrin. Anything with soy has MSG. Another problem with soy is 90 percent of the plants grow from GMO crops; this is a double whammy to our health.

Going back to the "no MSG" label, we know it is not true that there is no MSG present. Did the manufacturer try to hide this fact by printing the red "no" symbol "proving" that there is no MSG added? It is probably true that they did not "add" any MSG to the product; but in fact, it was already present within the ingredients. This is deceptive advertising to confuse and misinform the consumer—all this in order to get us to buy their product.

A closer look at the list shows that sugar, too, is present. As we have seen, sugar is addictive and promotes diabetes, obesity, and cancer. The ingredients listed on the label are from increasing to descending order of amounts of ingredient present in the product. Therefore, in the above seasoning salt example, salt is listed as the first ingredient because it comprises the largest amount of all ingredients contained in the product. Consequently, sugar is second so it must have a large amount in this salt product, but not as much as salt, and more than paprika. And so on. Having some knowledge about the dangers of certain ingredients, I would then return the product to the shelf and avoid purchasing it.

Here is the ingredients list of a popular muscle-building protein powder made from milk. The ingredients are taken directly from the manufacturer's website.

Ingredients:

Protein Blend (Calcium And Sodium Caseinate, Milk Protein Isolate, Whey Protein Hydrolysate, Whey Protein Concentrate, Lactoferrin, L-Glutamine, Taurine), Maltodextrin, Soluble Corn Fiber, Sunflower Oil, Canola Oil, Medium Chain Triglycerides, Crystalline Fructose, Di-Calcium Phosphate, Natural And Artificial Flavor, Less Than 1% Of: Potassium Bicarbonate, Inulin, Magnesium Oxide, Acesulfame-K, Potassium Bicarbonate, Soy Lecithin, Potassium Bicarbonate, Soy Lecithin, Sucralose, DL-Alpha Tocopheryl Acetate, Ascorbic Acid, Ferrous Fumarate, Vitamin A Palmitate, Niacinamide, Zinc Oxide, Copper Gluconate, Calcium Pantothenate, L-Carnitine, Cholecalciferol, Pyridoxine Hydrochloride, Thiamin Mononitrate, Riboflavin, Chromium Chloride, Folic Acid, Biotin, Potassium Iodide, Cyanocobalamin

Contains Ingredients Derived From Milk And Soy.

This Product Is Manufactured In A Facility That Processes Milk, Soy, Wheat And Eggs.

This product has some good ingredients, but the others scream out, loud and clear. Just look at the MSG components in the product! They include Caseinate, protein isolate, protein hydrolysate, protein concentrate, Maltodextrin, natural and artificial flavor, and soy lecithin. Also present are the harmful omega-6 oils, sunflower and canola. It has fructose, a sugar, and sucralose the artificial sweetener. It has thiamin Mononitrate; the thiamin is the vitamin b1, which is good, but it is attached to the nitrate preservative, which is not healthy. Lastly, it has soy on the list so we can assume it is probably a GMO. Looking at the total picture for ingredients, there are many additives that warrant considerable attention; and frankly, it is shocking the product promotes as a bodybuilding supplement.

To be fair in my reportage, I list below the ingredients of the protein powder I use, Orgain Organic Protein™, from the website of the manufacturer:

Ingredients:

Organic brown rice protein, organic chia seed, organic hemp protein, organic pea protein, organic creamer base (organic acacia gum, organic high oleic sunflower oil, organic inulin, organic rice dextrins, organic rice bran extract, organic rosemary extract), organic erythritol, organic cocoa, organic natural flavors, organic guar gum, organic xanthan gum, organic acacia gum, sea salt, organic stevia, monkfruit extract.

These are all organic ingredients, but a couple may cause concern. We see organic high oleic sunflower which, yes, is an omega-6 fat, however the high oleic acid component is the monounsaturated healthy fat found in olive oil. The next concern may be the organic xanthan gum. It is on the MSG list, but note that it is near the end of the ingredients list so the total amount if present would be small. Therefore, this product is a much better choice for protein powders. We may never be fully able to

CHAPTER TWO | THE HUMAN BODY

eliminate the bad foods and toxins, but we will try to minimize them, and maximize the good foods and nutrients.

We will look at one more ingredient label. This one is for a popular, quick noodle meal eaten by most college students.

Ingredients:

Noodle Ingredients: Enriched Wheat Flour (Wheat Flour, Niacin, Reduced Iron, Thiamine Mononitrate, Riboflavin, Folic Acid), Vegetable Oil (Contains One Or More Of The Following: Canola, Cottonseed, Palm), Preserved By TBHQ, Salt, Potassium Carbonate, Soy Sauce (Water, Wheat, Soybeans, Salt), Sodium Phosphate, Sodium Carbonate, Turmeric. Soup Base Ingredients: Salt, Chicken Fat, Monosodium Glutamate, Hydrolyzed Corn, Wheat And Soy Protein, Powdered Cooked Chicken, Sugar, Dehydrated Vegetables (Onion, Garlic, Chive), Dehydrated Soy Sauce (Wheat, Soybeans, Salt, Maltodextrin), Autolyzed Yeast Extract, Spices, Caramel Color, Natural And Artificial Flavors, Silicon Dioxide (Anti-Caking Agent), Lactose, Turmeric, Disodium Inosinate, Disodium Guanylate.

Not only are there numerous listings for ingredients that contain MSG, but the company was also brazen enough to actually list the "monosodium glutamate" by name. As if there was not enough of the excitotoxin flavor enhancer, they added more in its pure form. Also note that disodium inosinate and guanylate are included, which are always associated with MSG. No wonder it tastes good to the students that live off this meal; unfortunately, it is destined to create dementia in large numbers later in their lives.

We also find thiamine mononitrate and TBHQ, which are harmful preservatives. There is also sugar, omega-6 oils, caramel color dye, and probable GMO soy. Generally speaking, the more ingredients listed, the better the chance it contains harmful

HEALTHY BODY, HAPPY LIFE

ingredients. The products with the shortest ingredient list are very often, the healthiest.

Please read labels, be informed, and if you find a label to be misleading, contact the company. If more people tell the food manufacturers to put nutritious ingredients in the food, they will listen. Here is an example.

My wife and I were shopping at Costco, and I noticed the pricing sign stated that a common ranch salad dressing contained no MSG. I was curious to see if this was actually true. So, guess what? I read the label—which revealed it had soybean oil and soy flavors. This definitely has MSG, so the rack label was misleading the public.

I placed the two-pack dressing into the cart to show the store manager the misrepresentation. The checkout clerk summoned the manager, and I informed him of the error. He said he would look into it. The cashier asked me if I wanted to purchase the salad dressing—I politely told him "no thanks."

About one month later, we again were at the food club store and noticed the sign was still there. I asked my wife for a pen so I could scribble out the "no MSG" on the label. She admonishingly said "no!" to both the pen request and the act of defacing the sign. She said, "They have cameras and will take you away." Frankly, being hauled away was not a concern . . . But the false label was! Therefore, I went back to the cashier. The cashier gave me a number for Costco's corporate office in Washington State. The corporate person in charge of buying shelf products showed concern over the issue and provided the phone number of the salad dressing company representative to help resolve the issue.

After talking to the representative in California and explaining the problems with MSG and GMO soy—that they cause obesity, dementia, and breast cancer—she said she would talk to the appropriate management executives about this issue. I told her it was in the best interest of the company to make positive, healthy changes in the ingredients, because the public is more informed and making better health choices.

About two weeks later at Costco, I noticed the sign was changed; much to the relief of my wife, who did not have to see me carted off by security guards for taking a stand against mislabeling.

Buy Organic Foods

ONE SURE-FIRE way to avoid GMO foods and harmful pesticides is to buy organic foods whenever possible. The good news is that more grocery stores are realizing the need to provide fresh organic foods since the demand has greatly increased. The USDA has a certified organic department, which verifies if a farm is compliant with organic farming practices. The label to look for on food packages is this:

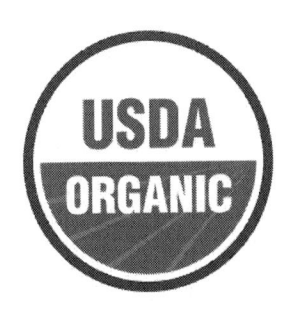

When it comes to foreign foods, be cautious if they claim to be organic. Research their organic claim further, as the policies and protocols for foreign food industries may not be the same as in the US. One country I do not buy food from is China. As a foreign country, they can grow their food as they please without much recourse. It is a known fact that the Chinese manufacturing industry can produce products cheaply, often because they pollute and sacrifice their environment in the process. Do you remember all the problems Beijing had with air pollution during the 2008 Summer Olympics? Chinese citizens have a higher incidence of lung cancer due to the air pollution. When in doubt as to the credibility of the food, buy American, with the "USDA Organic" label.

Another good practice is to buy locally from known farms. You will know if it is organic and fresh out of the fields. Food can travel from 1500 to 2000 miles and lose 40 percent of the nutritional value. The absolute best option is to grow your own food. This takes time and space, but you will have ultimate control over all aspects of production. Moreover, your children will learn good agricultural practices.

An important note: *organic foods and ingredients are grown without the use of harmful man-made pesticides, herbicides, fungicides, and they can't be GMOs. Acceptable organic practices allow spraying or exposure to "natural" pesticides, herbicides, and fungicides that appear on an "approved list" of acceptable agents. Animal products have not been given antibiotics or growth hormones and have been raised on "free range" farms or fed organic foods. This does not mean, however, that organic foods are free from all harmful additives even though they are organically derived. It is always best to read labels.*

CHAPTER TWO | THE HUMAN BODY

Eating at Restaurants

AVOID FAST-FOOD restaurants—the food is processed and flavored to sell fast . . . And kill slowly. Nevertheless, there may be times when you want to go to a good sit-down restaurant. If the restaurant posts the menu on-line, you can research the food selections beforehand. Determine if they are free from glutamate, excess refined sugar, omega-6 fats, or processed foods. If they do not have a website, you can ask the server when you get there.

We were at lunch one day, and the marinated chicken sandwich sounded good; but I was not sure about the marinade sauce—too many contain soy sauce. The server told me the marinade sauce was natural herb spices and extra virgin olive oil. I gave the restaurant extra kudos for being health conscience and the server a little extra tip.

References

The Cell: A Molecular Approach. 2nd edition. Cooper GM. Sunderland (MA): Sinauer Associates; 2000.

Molecular Cell Biology. 4th edition. Lodish H, Berk A, Zipursky SL, et al. New York: W. H. Freeman; 2000.

Blaylock, R.L., Blaylock wellness reports, Feb 2012.

Golomb, B., Evans, M.A., Am J Cardiovasc Drugs 2008; 8(6).

http://fitness.mercola.com/sites/fitness/archive/2013/06/28/intermittent-fasting-health-benefits.aspx?i_cid=cse-tbd-intermittent-fasting-content.

Blaylock, R.L., Excitotoxins: The Taste That Kills, Health Press, 1997.

Blaylock RL. Immunology primer for neurosurgeons and neurologists part I: Basic principles of immunology. Surg Neurol Int 2013;4:14.

Blaylock RL. Immunology primer for neurosurgeons and neurologists part 2: Innate brain immunity. Surg Neurol Int 2013;4:118.

Hudlický, Miloš (1996). *Reductions in Organic Chemistry*. Washington, D.C.: American Chemical Society.

http://www.vitalitymagazine.com/article/top-five-network-antioxidants/.

Blaylock, R.L., Blaylock wellness reports, May 2004.

Suzanne Humphries, MD, (2013) *Dissolving Illusions: Disease, Vaccines, and the forgotten History*. CreateSpace Independent Publishing Platform.

Blaylock, R.L., Blaylock wellness reports, May 2008.

Duggal T., MD, Am J Nephrol. 2013;38(2):174-8. doi: 10.1159/000354084. Epub 2013 Aug 6. *Anti Neutrophilcytoplasmic antibody vasculitis associated with influenza vaccination.* PMID 23941822.

Blaylock, R.L., Blaylock wellness reports, Feb 2011.

Cui, W.Y. and Li, M.D., J Neuroimmune Pharmacol 2010; 5: 479-88.

Noel Kingsbury. Hybrid: The History and Science of Plant Breeding. University of Chicago Press, Oct 15, 2009.

CHAPTER THREE
Nutritional Supplements, Vitamins and Minerals

If everyone ate organic, whole, raw foods full of nutrients, and took supplements, we would have an epidemic of health.

A deficiency of one vitamin can cause many illnesses. The addition of one vitamin can alleviate many illnesses.

~Andrew Saul, PhD

Nutrients from Plants

AS A CHRISTIAN and a scientist at heart, I believe God created a phenomenal creature called Homo sapiens. Mankind was given the precise molecular, cellular, tissue, and organ systems to perform many incredible functions—to survive and flourish. God also put humanity in a beautiful garden on the earth, full of fresh fruits and vegetables to nourish that wonderful creation. He provided nutraceuticals—plant-based nutrients to eat and thrive.

Picture yourself being in the Garden of Eden. What was there? Do you see dense trees and plants full of luscious food, with cool clear running water, and fresh air to breathe? In my mind's eye, I can picture this paradise.

This garden of fruits and vegetables was all they had for nourishment . . . But it was all they really needed. This was what I am calling the Garden of Eden Lifestyle, where humanity lived off the literal fruits of the land. God in his infinite wisdom, from the beginning of time, provided the human race the needed nourishment directly from the garden. However, in the mid-twentieth century, mankind in his infinite arrogance and ignorance thought food could be adulterated into something better. The results are in, and we now have more heart disease, diabetes, obesity, and cancer, all at ever-increasing rates.

Let's get back to that Garden of Eden Lifestyle and eat the nutritious foods that sustained life to the fullest.

Do you remember your mother telling you, as a child, to eat your vegetables if you wanted to grow up strong and healthy? What she said was very true—but how did she know that fruits and vegetables contain over 5,000 **phytonutrients** that improve our health and well-being? Phyto refers to plants, and phytonutrients are the nutrients within the plants. This is diet physiology at its best; just eat your vegetables and fruits and start nutritional healing of the body. *The good news, it is never too late!*

Unfortunately, over the years, vegetable consumption has lacked adequate quantities to prevent disease. However, if we want to live a healthier lifestyle, we need a paradigm shift in our lifestyle to include more of the nutrients from God's bounty—the natural world of healthy foods all around us. These awesome plants grew on earth for a reason; use them.

The recommended serving of vegetables is around eight to ten servings per day, or approximately three cups. For fruits, the amount is around two to three servings, or one cup. That's a lot of fruits and vegetables! Why so much?

When vegetables are cooked, the nutrients lose potency, so more consumption is required. In addition, chewing vegetables is usually only 20 percent efficient in breaking down the plant cellulose walls to release vital nutrients.

There are two ways to compensate for these problems. First, blanch (steam cook briefly) the raw vegetables so the nutrients are not lost but they can be easily chewed. Note that cruciferous vegetables (broccoli, cauliflower, Brussels sprouts, and kale) require blanching to inactivate the enzyme that inhibits the thyroxine hormone.

The second way to avoid eating mountains of fruits and vegetables and still benefit from the important phytonutrients is to "blenderize" them. Place them into the blender with water, and puree the contents. This mechanically breaks down the cell walls and allows for around 80 percent absorption of the nutrients.

One cup of blenderized vegetables and fruits is enough to satisfy the daily healthy requirement. Blenderizing will be examined in more detail in Chapter Six.

Another useful practice is to eat a greater variety of these plant foods so various phytonutrients can enrich the body. Blenderizing various vegetables and fruits will provide powerful antioxidant and anti-inflammatory properties, possibilities that are not as probable with pharmaceuticals (synthetic drugs).

Juicing is a good way to get more nutrients out of fruits and vegetables—but look at all the pulp left behind! Eating the pulp is good for the colon to help reduce colon cancer. Pulp also slows absorption of sugar and lowers insulin levels, thus reducing hunger.

Apply caution when eating fruits, especially if you have cancer. Fruits can have high levels of fructose (sugar), and it feeds cancer cells. Look at the glycemic index for fruits; raisins and figs are very high. Eat no more than one cup of fruits per day—less, if you have cancer.

Vitamins, Minerals, and Nutritional Supplements

WHY DO WE need additional nutrients? Frankly, in our American diet, we do not obtain the essential nutrients in quantities that will sustain us well.

Recall the story of the girl that ate dirt to get more iron. With poor diet choices, the brain will tell our body to continue eating in the attempt to acquire the necessary nutrients and we become obese in the process. With proper nourishment, while avoiding excess calories, we could avoid obesity and diseases as well.

Unfortunately this is even more difficult today because over the last century, the quality of fresh food has been decimated due to soil depletion, overproduction of crops, unsustainable farming practices, and the use of pesticides and herbicides.

We cannot assume we are getting all of the vitamins, minerals, and phytonutrients we need by eating varieties of fresh produce—

even when it is organically grown. *This is only accomplished through nutritional supplementation, which provides an efficient method for the body to obtain all the required nutrients to turn off the ghrelin hormone and turn on the leptin hormone—the second secret to a lean and healthy body.*

All of the vitamins, minerals, and supplements work synergistically in the human body. They are more powerful working together than the ability of any single component. If one chemical component for a particular metabolic process is missing, this negatively affects the entire chemical reaction cascade, which could prove catastrophic. If the quantity of an individual component is insufficient, it can also minimize the end metabolic result, leaving the person mal-nourished. Supplementing with nutrients is important; it will make up for missing or lacking metabolic components. Many of the biological nutrients will also aid in other various metabolic functions. For example, magnesium plays a role in over 300 different enzyme functions, while zinc is required in over 200.

Nutrients must have **bioavailability**, the ability to absorb into the body and assimilate into the cell or tissues at a level of concentration whereby it can produce the desired beneficial effects. Absorption by the gut does not necessarily mean it will get to the tissues or cells, but it is the first step to that possibility. The nutrient must get to the liver from the gut without interference by chemical alteration, which would render it into a non-usable form.

In the liver, nutrients metabolize into other products, some even more beneficial than before. These metabolites enter the blood stream and are transported to the rest of the body. This allows some nutrients to absorb into tissues at higher concentrations than in other tissues, which is why some nutrients

HEALTHY BODY, HAPPY LIFE

are more critical for the health of certain organs and tissues and where the specific nutrient demand is greater.

Nutrients come in various forms: tablet, capsule, and soft gels. The capsule can be made from animal fat, which is not as desirable, since it can contain unwanted animal contaminants (antibiotics, pesticides, and chemicals); or from vegetarian and vegan materials, which is the better choice. The soft gels are capsules that contain a liquid, usually oil. For best bioavailability, soft gels are the preferred vessel because they already have nutrients dissolved in oil for the best absorption. Moreover, the vegetarian or vegan capsule is readily broken down, releasing the contents. The tablet is the third best option; most are broken down in the gut but not always, depending upon the binding agents. In general, powdered supplements or liquids are best because they come from the natural source in the most functional form.

For those having difficulty swallowing supplements, I have found that it is best to divide them up into what I call "sinkers" and "floaters". Sinkers are usually tablets and soft gels that will sink in water. Floaters are generally the capsules that float. For sinkers, take a half mouth full of water, tip your head back to drop them in, purse your lips (pucker) to remove excess air inside your mouth by pushing the water forward, close your lips, and take a big swallow to consume the entire contents in your mouth at once.

For the floaters, take a half mouth full of water, tip your head back to drop in the supplements, purse the lips to remove excess air, and close your lips—but now dip your chin down before you take a big swallow. This allows the floaters to rise to the back of your throat making it easier to swallow. Start with one, or a few of each, until you get the process down. Bet you didn't think taking supplements would be this much fun, right?

CHAPTER THREE | NUTRITIONAL SUPPLEMENTS

Supplements also need to have the correct dosage to be most effective. The great news for supplements is that the maximum toxic dose is usually very high—and mostly not even achievable. The few exceptions are explained in the list of supplements below.

Supplements have a high safety record when compared to prescription medications. Nevertheless, if you take prescription medications, talk to your pharmacist to rule out any possible harmful interactions with supplements. The proper use of supplements can reduce the need for the much more expensive pharmaceutical drugs, along with a reduction of their harmful side effects.

Many supplements will treat the "cause" of a condition or disorder, whereas many drugs will just mask the problem—treating symptoms—and not solve the underlying cause. Here are some informative statistics. From a study involving a 23-year span, ten people died from overdosing with supplements. How does this compare with modern medicine and the use of prescription medications?

In our current medical delivery system, 39,000 deaths per year are due to unnecessary surgery; 80,000 deaths per year are from nosocomial infections (caused by *infections obtained in the hospital environment*); and 106,000 deaths per year are from adverse prescription drug interactions, even though they were taken as prescribed. The bottom line is at least 225,000 deaths per year result from the processes of modern medicine. If you only look at the number of deaths due to adverse drug reactions—106,000 per year—and multiply that by the 23 years the supplement study covered, we get just under 2.5 million total deaths from prescription drugs. These were from side effects and drug interactions while taken as directed. Compare this to the ten deaths from supplements, and we immediately see which has the better record of accomplishment. Therefore, if a supplement could diminish or prevent a disease, it would be better to start there, and enjoy the better safety record.

We do not need Big Pharma to create the "miracle drug" to solve all our health problems—because frankly, they can't produce a "miracle drug" that has no side effects; and synthetic pharmaceuticals often do not cure the problem, but just mask the symptoms.

God's pharmacy created all the body's necessary miracle nutrients—called food: wholesome, natural, organic, nutritious fruits and vegetables. Not the processed, synthetic junk food we think is good for us, which is actually making us all sick. All while, these companies are making huge profits—at the expense of our health. Medical science is continually discovering how natural foods, supplements, and minerals are preventing and even curing many diseases. In addition, a good diet and natural supplements help protect us from the side effects of many prescription drugs and allow many patients to use much lower doses of drugs.

Supplements are also far less expensive than prescription medications, mainly because expensive research is required to develop such prescription drugs. With supplements, God and the natural world have done the research for us—and without a price tag! Moreover, with supplements, most side effects have proven beneficial. If you listen to the commercial ads from drug companies, at the end you hear all the negative side effects of the expensive prescription medicines. They are often crammed into the last few seconds of the ad, which makes it nearly impossible to decipher by the normal human ear! Why would you want to subject yourself to the possibility of harmful side effects, or even death? Would you rather take prescription drugs with many known and proven horrendous side effects, or would you rather take God's food and supplements, with known and proven numerous healthy crossover benefits? Choose wisely for your health most desperately depends on it.

Numerous studies have researched the pros and cons of supplements. Many listed on the internet paint them in a negative light. Decide for yourself if the researcher or the study may be biased or compromised. Many studies that purport the ineffectiveness of certain supplements may have applied their tests only to supplements with either poor bioavailability, or without the important context of testing it with other supplements. Remember that nutrients are synergistic and work best together, hence, it seems logical to avoid testing supplements in isolation. Other studies may report no health benefit from a supplement, but looking at the data would suggest nothing would have worked to prove their point, not even a prescription drug. Then we must look at the scientists or company behind the study. Remember when tobacco companies performed studies and concluded smoking does not increase the risk of lung cancer? We all know better now. The lesson here is, always check your sources!

In my opinion, I have found contradictory and misleading information about supplements on Wikipedia, a popular internet information website, which may get advertising revenues from pharmaceutical companies. I like the website for other topics and think it is a good source for general descriptions. However, for better, detailed, and non-biased information about supplements, look at other, more reliable and scientifically vetted sources, including scientific journals.

Supplements work to prevent disease and alleviate illnesses, but some may require long-term use to be most effective. It took a long time for the body to degrade into a disease state, and thus, it will surely take time to reverse that course. *Supplements work best when combined with a healthy diet, exercise, reduced stress, avoidance of toxic chemicals, and good sleep.* These are the keys to good health espoused throughout this book.

It is far easier to prevent disease with good nutrition and proper use of supplements than to cure a disease once it presents itself in the body. As Ben Franklin said, "An ounce of prevention is worth a pound of cure." That absolutely remains true today and perhaps more than ever.

We will now look at vitamins.

Vitamins

A VITAMIN IS a necessary organic compound, but one that can't be synthesized in our body: it must be obtained through our diet or through supplementation. The word **vitamin** stands for vital amine, as coined by Kazimierz Funk, a Polish biochemist, in 1911. He thought they were vital—which is true—and were an organic group of compounds called amines—which is partially true. In fact, some are amines, but others are not. Vitamins are required for many different bodily chemical reactions. A letter designates the group, which classifies them with similar chemical make-up and therefore their concomitant functions. While vitamins are required in small quantities, their absence can cause enormous health problems.

We will take a closer look at each one. Most of these vitamins will be part of our regimen used to protect the body and promote health. Use the following as a reference guide, as needed.

Vitamin A includes a group known as carotenoids, which includes beta-carotene (from carrots) and helps with eyesight. Another carotenoid is lycopene, found in tomatoes and converts into Vitamin A. Astaxanthin is a carotenoid, but fails to transform into vitamin A; it is a powerful antioxidant. Vitamin A has multiple functions: it is important for growth and development, for the maintenance of the immune system, and for good vision. We ingest it from many leafy, colorful vegetables.

Vitamin B refers to the B complex of vitamins, which consist of eight main subgroups that are water-soluble and play important roles in cell metabolism. They function as precursors for enzyme cofactors, as well as in DNA repair. This is the largest group of vitamins, and each B vitamin is chemically distinct, as described here:

B1 (thiamine)—involved in many cellular processes and metabolism. A deficiency is associated with beriberi, which involves weight loss, pain, and weakness of the limbs.

B2 (riboflavin)—the central component of cofactors for enzyme reactions. It turns urine yellow.

B3 (niacin or niacinamide)—the better functional form is niacinamide, which does not cause facial flushing. It aids in the citric acid cycle as a cofactor to produce ATP energy in mitochondria.

B5 (pantothenic acid)—used to synthesize coenzyme-A and metabolize proteins, carbohydrates, and fat.

B6 (pyridoxine, pyridoxal, or pyridoxamine)—serves as a cofactor in many enzymatic reaction.

B7 (biotin)—a metabolic coenzyme that must be present in equal amounts with other B vitamins for absorption by the body.

B9 (folic acid or folate)—the best functional form is methyl folate. It will synthesize and repair DNA and acts as a cofactor. It aids cell division and growth, especially in infants.

B12 (cobalamin)—methylcoalamin is the best functional form. It is used to treat diabetic neuropathy and amyotrophic lateral sclerosis (ALS—Lou Gehrig's disease).

Many B vitamins work together to impede many diseases and cancers. Deficiencies of B vitamins are associated with high levels of homocysteine, a metabolic breakdown product associated with inflammation. Homocysteine levels also increase naturally with age. Sources of vitamin B are legumes (beans), whole grains, potatoes, bananas, and meat.

Vitamin C is an essential nutrient that humans can't synthesize in the body; we get it quite readily from citrus fruits and meat. It functions in the body as ascorbic acid, or as the salt or ionic form, ascorbate. The best bioavailable form is magnesium ascorbate, which means we can get magnesium along with it.

Vitamin C is a water-soluble cofactor in many enzymatic and metabolic reactions and has anti-inflammatory as well as antioxidant properties. Vitamin C works to protect the cells of the body in the aqueous environment (cytosol), while other, fat-soluble, antioxidants (CoQ10/vitamin E) protect the cells of the body in the organic phase environment, or cell membranes.

Take vitamin C on an empty stomach, otherwise it will facilitate iron absorption by the body; excess absorbed iron is carcinogenic since the salt or ionic form is a free radical. Iron also promotes bacterial and viral infections, atherosclerosis, and brain degeneration. Also, *do not take vitamin B12 along with vitamin C, as vitamin C will degrade the B12 and make it less effective.*

Vitamin C promotes collagen strength of connective tissue, the underlying matrix of most tissues. Collagen supports all organs and blood vessel integrity. A deficiency can lead to swelling of the ankles, varicose veins (seen in the elderly because they have a harder time absorbing vitamin C), hemorrhoids, aneurysms, and loose hanging skin. Collagen is also important as the bone matrix for repair and healing, as well as general wound healing. Smoking causes a vitamin C deficiency and explains the wrinkled, aged skin, associated with vascular diseases, and cancer. Also, do not cook with vitamin C, as heat will break it down into a non-functional form.

Vitamin C protects the heart. It reduces atherosclerosis and thus reduces heart attacks and strokes. Vitamin C can also relax blood vessels and thus lower blood pressure. Vitamin C also protects the brain, which has the highest vitamin C concentration levels. This helps reduce oxidative stress and inflammation.

Vitamin D is a neurohormone that performs many functions. The active form is vitamin D3 (cholecalciferol) and the skin synthesizes it by utilizing UVB (ultraviolet B) sunlight. UVB is readily absorbed by the ozone layer, so the sun must be 45 degrees or higher for the rays to penetrate the atmosphere to be effective. Get exposure on as much of your body as possible for up to one hour, or until pink; but avoid burning. If you plan on longer sun exposure, apply a sunscreen, but don't use one with harsh chemicals that create their own toxic problems.

Sunscreens with PABA (para-aminobenzoic acid—a preservative), Oxybenzone, and dioxybenzone are potent free-radical generators that cause cancer. Use one with 4.5% zinc oxide, or stay in the shade. If you go to a tanning salon, use beds that have UVB lamps, not the UVA (ultra violet A) lamps that have the deeper penetrating UV light. Again, do not burn yourself and stop after you are a little pink.

Vitamin D3 helps build strong bones by promoting calcium absorption; prevents cancer (especially melanoma) and heart disease; aids in cellular function, assists in brain development (helps prevent autism) and promotes immunity. The amount of vitamin D3 present is directly proportional to immunity—the more vitamin D3 one has, the better their immunity.

Vitamin D3 has a binding protein, called **Gc protein** (Globulin component protein), that is the molecular carrier for vitamin D3 in the blood. Gc protein plays a major role in protection from infections since it is the precursor of **MAF** (macrophage activating factor), which activates the macrophages in cellular immunity. The macrophages phagocytize (gobble up) infection causing microbes, and direct other immune cells during the invasion.

During infection or a developing cancer, the Gc protein converts into MAF, which recruits an army of macrophages to battle the foreign invaders. However, within the cell walls of bacteria, viruses, fungi, and cancer cells there is an enzyme called **nagalase** (N-acetlygalactosaminidase), which prevents MAF from being converted from Gc protein, thereby disarming the immune system. Researchers are developing ways to neutralize nagalase and enhance MAF production. Another way to over-power nagalase is to promote more MAF by supplementing with vitamin D3, to force the production of more immune stimulators.

Cancer patients, and those with severe infections, have high levels of nagalase and low levels of MAF; this allows the cancer and infection to evade the immune system. Infusion of MAF in prostate, colorectal, and breast cancer patients, has had great results in fighting cancer, with few side effects. The changing prognosis of disease or its treatment will influence nagalase blood levels. Cancer growth and its spread within the body increase nagalase levels, which are detectable; healthy people do not have nagalase present in their body.

Cancer cells also produce nagalase, which will elevate blood levels and inhibit cellular immunity. Because there is a nagalase blood test to determine blood levels, it is possible to measure nagalase levels in response to cancer treatment, which will indicate if the treatment is working.

GcMAF also inhibits angiogenesis, a powerful aid to fight cancer. Angiogenesis is the induction of new blood vessels by the cancer cells that supply nutrients to the cancer tumor. Since GcMAF is the D3 carrier protein, higher levels of D3, through supplementation or sun exposure, promote more production of GcMAF. This is how vitamin D3 enhances immunity.

Over the years, the incidence of melanoma cancer has increased, not decreased, even though more sunscreen is in use today. One can conclude then that it is not due to sun over-exposure, but actually due to the lack of sunlight to generate appropriate levels of vitamin D3. People living in the more northern latitudes, where there is less ultraviolet B (UVB) ambient light, and/or in places where people use too much sunscreen, there is a higher incidence of melanoma cancer. The lack of vitamin D3 production decreases the immune capability of the skin to inhibit and slow melanoma occurrence.

Vitamin D3 is vital for immunity to inhibit or kill many viruses, bacteria, and fungi. This explains why viruses are less severe near the equator (more UVB light), and that the elderly, who are more vitamin D3 deficient, have more severe flu attacks. Viruses also have the nagalase enzyme, on the viral envelope protein coat, and this is why it can be difficult for our immune system to eradicate the flu virus.

A vitamin D3 deficiency encourages seizures due to over-activity in brain tissues that causes free radicals and promotes the excitotoxicity process. The deficiency also occurs in autoimmune disorders such as multiple sclerosis and rheumatoid arthritis: vitamin D3 supplementation can lessen their symptoms.

Vitamin D3 deficiency causes SAD (seasonal affective disorder), due to lack to light during the winter months. SAD is associated with carbohydrate cravings (for hibernation and fat accumulation mode), daytime sleepiness, lack of energy, and depression. Have you ever wondered why in the springtime, after a long dark winter, that on the first beautiful sunny day, people are cheerful and exuberant? They are finally generating much-needed vitamin D3.

When we get vitamin D3 naturally from the sun, it can be as much as 40,000 IU's (international units) per day. The harmful doses are extremely high and are in the hundreds of thousands to be toxic. RDA recommendations are only 400 IU's per day, but this is not enough. Children should take 1,000 IU's per day, young adults 2,000 IU's per day, and adults 5,000 IU's per day. Pregnant moms also need vitamin D3 to aid in fetal brain development. Those with cancer or autoimmune disorders should take between 5,000-10,000 IU's per day.

Vitamin E consists of lipid-soluble compounds, which contain two groups called tocopherols and tocotrienols. There are five subgroups: alpha, beta, delta, gamma, and epsilon. They are the major antioxidant and anti-inflammatory components in the fat-soluble part of the cell. Gamma tocopherol is an anti-inflammatory, which helps prevent cancer. Alpha tocopherols are antioxidants and prevent oxidation of LDL cholesterol in brain cell membranes. Tocotrienols are powerful antioxidants, which promote brain health and prevent brain cancer.

Dry E is the water-soluble form of vitamin E for better absorption and bioavailability. Together with selenium, they boost immunity. The source of vitamin E is plant oils and vegetables.

Vitamin K is a fat-soluble group the body needs to make blood-clotting proteins and proteins used to bind calcium in bone and tissues. Without vitamin K, uncontrolled bleeding would occur, and we would have weaker bones. There are two main subgroups: vitamin K1, and vitamin K2. Vitamin K1 transforms into vitamin K2, which is the active form.

Vitamin P (Bioflavonoids) was a classification in the mid 1930's through early 1950's, but the vitamin P designation discontinued and became bioflavonoids. They are a class of plant *secondary* nutrients, which are not directly involved with our growth or development. However, the absence of them could adversely affect our health and long-term survival. An example is curcumin, the turmeric spice that decreases inflammation. Note that deficiencies of plant *primary* nutrients result in sure death, as our bodies require them to perform specific biological functions. An example of a primary plant nutrient is vitamin C, where a deficiency leads to scurvy and then one's demise.

Bioflavonoids aid plants in defense from predators and have other secondary roles. Found in many plant species, these secondary nutrients are used by people as medicines, flavorings, and recreational drugs.

Many bioflavonoids metabolize in the gut by probiotics that convert them into better forms of nutrients; and they transform in the liver into forms the body can readily use. Cooking with high heat can destroy bioflavonoids so cook them at lower temperatures.

Many of the 5,000 bioflavonoids are not available in supplement form, so you must eat them directly. A good diet will include these nutritious foods.

One bioflavonoid, ellagic acid, is of particular importance as it inhibits and kills cancer cells. It is found in many fruits, particularly berries (strawberries, raspberries, blueberries, and blackberries), and nuts. Ellagic acid prevents cancer development and growth by inhibiting carcinogens from binding to healthy cell DNA and thus inhibiting DNA mutations, which would lead to

CHAPTER THREE | NUTRITIONAL SUPPLEMENTS

cancer cells. It also causes cancer cell death in tumors.

The following list of **bioflavonoid subgroups** includes some foods that contain them, but the food lists are not exhaustive. We will include many of these in the vegetables/fruits smoothie described in Chapter Six, to insure we obtain the benefit of the vast goodness of these phytonutrients.

Anthocyanins—berries, purple cabbage, fruits with purple, red, or blue color, and grapes

Apigenin—carrots, celery, parsley

Caffeic acid—apricots, apples, blueberries, plums, and tomatoes

Catechin—grapes, tea, and red wine

Chlorogenic acid—McIntosh apples, blueberries, eggplant, and tomato skin

Curcumin—turmeric spice

Ellagic acid (ellagitannins)—pomegranates, raspberries, strawberries, and walnuts

Epicatechins—Hawthorn, and tea (especially white and green)

Epigallocatechin gallate—black and red currents, peaches, and tea (white/green)

Ferulic acid—some fruits and peppers

Hesperidin—black currants, grapefruit, and oranges

Kaempferol—broccoli, cherries, black currants, kale, onions, strawberries, tea, and turnip greens

Luteolin—artichokes, carrots, celery, and lettuce

Myricetin—broad beans, grapes, teas, and red wine

Naringenin—grapefruit, and oranges

Nobiletin—tangerines

Quercetin—cranberries, apples, cilantro, and onions

Tangeretin—tangerines

Minerals

DIETARY MINERALS ARE chemical elements needed for biological processes. Many are cofactors that catalyze cellular metabolism. The seven major dietary elements are calcium, phosphorus, potassium, sulfur, sodium, chlorine, and magnesium. Important trace elements are selenium, zinc, iron, iodine, bromine, copper, manganese, and molybdenum; and ultra-trace elements are boron and chromium.

Fortunately, a dietary supplement contains all these important minerals. It's called Concentrace® Trace Mineral Drops. We will see in Chapter Six how it is added to our regimen of a healthy diet. Now let's look at those minerals important to our quest for better health.

Calcium is the most abundant element found mainly in bones. In addition, it is also an important cell-signaling messenger in the body. The mitochondria regulate the amount of calcium taken into the cell through calcium channels in the membrane. There are optimal calcium levels, and when exceeded, will cause cellular death. This is what happens with aging: the mitochondria become inefficient and calcium regulation fails. This can disrupt many cell protein synthesis processes, especially in the brain.

To avoid excess calcium, restrict the dose to no more than 500 mg per day; and always use magnesium and vitamin D3 along with it (this is part of the synergistic effect). Vitamin D3 promotes the uptake of calcium into bones and reduces cancer risk, while magnesium helps prevent the excess blood calcium from building up in atherosclerotic plaque in the arteries and arthritic joints.

Excess calcium is associated with cancer growth, migraines, strokes, heart attacks, brain injury, immune dysfunctions, and

CHAPTER THREE | NUTRITIONAL SUPPLEMENTS

diabetes. Taking vitamin D3 regulates calcium and improves bone health and heart muscle function. The cause of osteoporosis is not a calcium deficiency, but from a deficiency in vitamin D3. Without enough Vitamin D3 to promote calcium uptake, not enough absorbs into bone.

Hyper-parathyroidism causes increased blood levels of calcium, with the breakdown of bone. Pregnant mothers have decreased calcium levels due to the developing fetal calcium requirements, creating a deficiency in moms' calcium. People with hyper-parathyroidism and pregnant mothers are at risk for low calcium; monitor closely for levels of calcium, vitamin D3, and magnesium.

Magnesium is an essential element that aids in over 300 biological processes and acts as both an anti-inflammatory and antioxidant agent. Unfortunately, 75 percent of people are deficient in magnesium and do not even know it. The *routine* blood test for magnesium assesses the amount in circulating blood; however, only 1 percent circulates in the blood, so this test doesn't give an adequate representation of true cellular levels. An *RBC (red blood cell) essential mineral test* will determine the amount of magnesium absorbed by the red blood cells and is representative of magnesium levels for all tissues. Most labs can perform the test.

Magnesium stops inflammation by inhibiting the calcium-triggered inflammation pathways in cells and prevents calcium build-up in atherosclerosis. Magnesium reduces intra-vascular blood clotting and guards the heart against attacks, failure, arrhythmias, and muscle degeneration, all by decreasing inflammatory cytokines in the muscle. Magnesium competes with and blocks glutamate receptors that cause excitotoxicity in the heart, which would otherwise cause arrhythmias.

The same glutamate receptors in the heart are also in the brain, and magnesium will block them from causing chronic brain excitotoxicity. Thus, it will regulate brain neurotransmitter activity and help alleviate pain (especially migraine headaches), seizures, and brain injury leading to dementia.

An American diet comprised of red meat, omega-6 fats, sugar, insufficient amounts of fruits/vegetables, and excessive soda pop depletes the body of magnesium; it gets worse as we age. Anti-hypertensives, statins, and birth control pills deplete the body of magnesium as well—supplementation will help in all cases.

Excessive doses of magnesium can cause diarrhea, but under normal doses this does not occur unless other medications also promote diarrhea. To eliminate diarrhea, take time-released magnesium supplements. Use magnesium in the form of magnesium malate or magnesium citrate since these have better bioavailability than magnesium oxide, which is poorly absorbed.

If you need elective surgery, boost your magnesium intake starting from two months before surgery, especially if you have low RBC essential mineral levels. It slowly absorbs into the body and takes extra time to reach therapeutic levels. Magnesium helps to counter the long-term effects of general anesthetics. It also reduces post-operative pain and promotes healing.

Selenium is a trace element that functions with glutathione peroxidase, an enzyme, to support glutathione in antioxidation—remember glutathione is a very important liver antioxidant. Selenium helps prevent chronic inflammation from free radicals and thus helps decrease brain excitotoxicity. It also aids in the conversion of the inactive thyroid hormone T4 into the active T3 form.

CHAPTER THREE | NUTRITIONAL SUPPLEMENTS

Zinc is another trace element, and it aids in over 200 metabolic reactions. Like magnesium, it is an ion of similar size and charge. Zinc is effective in helping to control infections and aids the immune system.

Magnesium, selenium, and zinc assist the five main antioxidants of the body, which are part of the antioxidant network.

Iron is bound in red blood cells, which transports oxygen from the lungs to the cells for oxidative metabolism. It aids in the generation of cell energy and is a cofactor in many enzymatic biological processes. The body requires a delicate balance to maintain healthy iron levels. Low iron levels can cause fatigue as well as heart failure from low oxygen levels, rapid aging from mitochondrial failure (also due to low oxygen), and susceptibility to many diseases.

However, high iron levels are dangerous too. It can cause rapid aging of tissues from oxidative stress, neurodegenerative disorders (such as Alzheimer's) from excitotoxicity, atherosclerosis via free radicals and lipid peroxidation (oxidation of omega-6 fats and LDL cholesterol) that leads to heart attacks and strokes, diabetes, and higher cancer risk from even higher free radical levels. There is a definite balance required, but higher levels are worse than lower levels.

Have your iron levels checked. Lab test results for iron should be in the low to middle normal range. A complete iron panel measures free iron, transferrin levels, transferrin saturation, and ferritin levels.

Free iron, in the ionic state, is extremely toxic and highly reactive, so binding to a carrier protein within the body prevents free radicals, inflammation, and cancer. Red meat is high in iron and best eaten with plenty of vegetables to bind the excess. Since vitamin C absorbs iron, it is best to take the vitamin between meals to prevent excessive iron absorption.

Excess iron can make cancers grow faster and become more invasive. High levels of iron in a person with a serious infection can make the infection worse or even fatal. All this is because bacteria, viruses, and cancer need iron in the DNA replication process to rapidly divide and grow.

Pre-menopausal women should take multivitamins with iron, since their body lacks iron due to menses. However, post-menopausal women, and most men, should take multivitamins without iron because enough will be absorbed in the diet. Post-menopausal women have more fatal heart attacks and strokes because their body's demand for iron is less, but they still consume an excessive amount, which promotes the atherosclerosis.

Nutritional Supplements

DIETARY SUPPLEMENTS PROVIDE nutrients to people who may not obtain the proper amount through food. There are thousands of supplements available, with the most common one consumed as the multivitamin. One pharmaceutical company produced a television commercial for their multivitamin that ran in the spring of 2016. The commercial stated, "Americans, 57 percent of us try to exercise regularly, 83 percent try to eat healthy, yet up to 90 percent of us fall short in getting key nutrients from food alone. Let's do more together." Their research led them to acknowledge that food does not provide enough nutrition for 90 percent of the population; that is significant. However, taking a multivitamin alone is not enough to reverse the problem. Multivitamins are a great start, but the nutrients in them are too few and their dosages too low for adequate protection.

Both a nutritious diet and supplements are important for a healthy body. Since most diets do not contain all the nutrients our bodies need, an alternate source is required. After many years with inadequate supplies of essential nutrients, the body begins to show signs of disease, disorders, and even cancers, as evidenced by the ever-increasing rates of ill health today. Most of the time it takes decades of chronic inflammation for the body to get to that point; so it makes sense that taking supplements means it will take time to reverse the damage. If we put off eating healthy foods and taking supplements, our day of better health may never arrive.

The power of supplements is synergy; most have cross-reactive benefits to alleviate multiple conditions. Taking various supplements works together to provide all the metabolic processes the body needs, to survive and to thrive. Taking just one supplement because it is the latest fad may not result in visible improvement, only because another necessary nutrient may be lacking, which hinders completion of the biological chemical process.

Always buy pharmaceutical grade supplements. They must pass a more strict manufacturing process, and assure better quality and bioavailability. Put the supplements in the refrigerator, they will last longer; especially the soft gels, which contain oil. Heat and light can oxidize the oil, making it rancid and ineffective. If the supplement bottle comes with an oxygen absorber, keep it inside to prevent oxidation as well.

How do we know when we have eaten enough nutritious food and taken the right supplements to get all the vital nutrients our bodies need? Unless you have routine blood tests to evaluate nutrient levels, you will never know for sure scientifically—except that you will look good and feel even better! It is better to err on the side of caution and consume enough nutrients and supplements since there is little chance to exceed maximum amounts.

The recommended regimen in this book provides safe guidelines; and any excesses the body cannot use, are excreted. Probabilities are much higher that we are lacking many nutrients and could use a boost. Remember 75 percent of Americans are deficient in magnesium and do not even know it.

Many chronic health problems originate from nutrient deficiencies in a poor diet. Too often, in order to treat the ailment, the healthcare provider will prescribe a drug to mask the symptoms instead of curing the nutrient deficiency with supplements. Unfortunately, most physicians receive very little instruction on the benefits of nutrition and supplements. In my own case, in dental school, the studies on supplementation were severely lacking.

Our beautifully designed body responds to natural healing from food nutrients. The nourishing molecules help our body repair, revitalize, and heal itself the way God intended—by using God's pharmacy, found only in nature.

Supplements are usually extracts, concentrated forms of natural molecules found in food. Our body knows how to absorb and use them in a balanced way, not only to relieve symptoms, but also to cure the cause of disease. In addition, as if that wasn't awesome enough, there are far fewer side effects than with prescription drugs, and the supplements cost far less.

The following list of supplements describes the ones most

advantageous if taken regularly, along with their unique benefits. There are thousands of nutrients, but these are the most crucial.

These supplements are included in our regimen seen in Chapter Six to help develop a leaner, stronger body. Along your life's journey, you may find the need for additional supplements to add to this list, but this is a great starting point.

The list of most beneficial supplements.

The intent is that you do not need to commit this information to memory, but rather use it as a reference. View the information for a better understanding of the significance and enormous crossover benefits from the supplements. They are in alphabetical order for easier referencing, accompanied by the suggested single dose if applicable.

Aged Garlic Extract results from aging raw garlic in 20 percent ethanol, for 20 months. This process breaks down the enzyme allicin, but releases S-allylmercaptocysteine, allixin, and selenium—three antioxidants that fight off atherosclerosis. Aged garlic also dissolves blood clots and thins blood, which is important for diabetics who have a high incidence of heart attacks and strokes due to clots forming from atherosclerotic plaques.

Aged garlic extract lowers blood pressure by relaxing blood vessels, reduces arrhythmias, has antibacterial/fungal/viral properties, increases good HDL cholesterol, prevents oxidation of bad LDL cholesterol, improves immunity, and reduces blood sugar in diabetics. Aged garlic is a powerful antioxidant that performs better against atherosclerosis than statins. It protects the brain from excitotoxins like mercury, by binding and removing it from the body, and has anti-cancer effects.

Garlic starts to work within three hours and lasts four to six hours. Heating destroys the allicin enzyme, so be mindful during cooking. Garlic is toxic in the 20,000+ mg doses, which is extremely high.

Alpha Lipoic Acid is also called just lipoic acid; they are the same acid. As a universal powerful antioxidant, it restores antioxidant power to other antioxidants like vitamin C and vitamin E. Even when oxidized, it will still keep the other antioxidants in their reduced, protective state.

Alpha lipoic acid has many benefits for diabetes since it lowers blood sugar by improving cellular uptake of glucose (especially in muscle cells) by increasing insulin sensitivity. It promotes more cell energy, fights peripheral neuropathy that causes painful and tingling limbs, and aids metabolism by protecting and repairing mitochondria from aging.

Alpha lipoic acid also binds and removes toxic metals like mercury and excess iron. It fights radiation damage from mammograms, CT, and PET scans. It helps in the after-effects of strokes by reducing excitotoxins in the brain. Alpha lipoic acid aids in treating burning mouth syndrome, helps liver cells detoxify the body by increasing liver glutathione levels (another powerful antioxidant), speeds wound healing, fights neurodegenerative disorders (Alzheimer's, dementia, etc.), and helps with hypertension. This is a very versatile compound and very protective.

Due to the ability to increase glucose uptake in the cells, exercise caution for those susceptible to reactive hypoglycemia. This condition involves excessive insulin release during a high glycemic meal, which causes a rebound low blood sugar level (hypoglycemia) that can be dangerous and even fatal.

Alpha lipoic acid may deplete vitamin B7 (biotin), and vitamin B12 (methylcobalamin) levels so they need to be taken along with lipoic acid. Also, note that R-lipoic acid is the more biofunctional form of alpha lipoic acid, so limit its dose to 50 mg to prevent hypoglycemia; but alpha lipoic acid at 250 mg is still a good option.

Astaxanthin is a carotenoid and a powerful antioxidant that reduces free radicals. It calms an inflammatory cytokine storm to lessen the immune response; thus, it is also an anti-inflammatory agent. It may help slow cellular aging by modulating the insulin-signaling pathway, which would otherwise lead to oxidative stress from excessive free radicals produced by mitochondria during glucose metabolism.

Beta 1,3/1,6 Glucan boosts cell-mediated immunity by increasing the number of white blood cells that gobble up (phagocytize) invading organisms like bacteria and viruses. In addition to fighting infections, it helps fight cancer by destroying cancer cells and protects from radiation damage during mammograms, CT, and PET scans. Take one daily, for two to three weeks during an active infection, or before an upcoming surgery, and then continue for one week afterwards. Take a maintenance dose of one per week to ward off infections, flu, and cancer.

Borage Oil comes from Borage seeds, which has a high concentration of GLA (gamma linolenic acid) at 28 percent. Gamma Linolenic Acid derives from Linoleic acid (a healthy omega-6 fat) and reduces inflammation, plus the growth and spread of cancer. GLA inserts itself into cancer cell membranes, where it transforms into DGLA (dihomo gamma linolenic acid) from the addition of two carbons onto the GLA fatty acid chain.

DGLA produces free radicals and lipid peroxidation products *only within the cancer cell*, but *not in normal host cells*. Thus, oxidation only occurs within the cancer cells and causes their destruction.

Inflammation is the immune response to deal with invasion of foreign bodies. The immune system COX (cyclooxygenase) enzyme promotes prostaglandins, which invoke an inflammatory response. The COX enzyme changes DGLA into the inflammatory PGE1 (prostaglandin 1) which induces inflammation and thus kills only cancer cells. Note that Vitamin E and NSAID's (non-steroidal anti-inflammatory drugs, like ibuprofen) will block the COX enzyme and prevent the DGLA from killing cancer cells. Therefore, suspend Vitamin E supplements and NSAID's while taking GLA for active cancer treatment, so they do not inhibit the free radical killing of the cancer cells.

DGLA is better than chemotherapy drugs because chemotherapy causes free radicals and lipid peroxidation in both cancer and normal cells, while DGLA only attacks cancer cells. DGLA also, does not develop multidrug resistance, as chemotherapeutic agents so commonly do. Borage can be used alone or even with chemo agents.

GLA will also improve moisture and mucous membranes. It can help prevent dry eyes and mouth.

Carnitine comes in two major forms: L-carnitine and acetyl-L-carnitine.

L-carnitine is better for weight loss, building muscle mass and athletic endurance. It mobilizes the long-chained fatty acids into the mitochondria for energy use, especially when combined with diet and exercise.

Acetyl-L-carnitine passes the blood-brain barrier and

provides better brain benefits, such as increased cellular energy via mitochondrial enhanced production. It also has an acetyl substrate for acetylcholine synthesis, a neurotransmitter that helps in brain and heart nerve conduction.

Mitochondrial function benefits by acetyl-L-carnitine. It supplies cells with energy and regulates calcium levels in the cells—an excess of calcium can cause cell death. Aging is very dependent upon mitochondrial function and efficiency, especially in the heart and brain. Failing mitochondria can lead to higher levels of free radicals that cause excitotoxicity, or over-activation of the brain immune system (microglia) due to increased glutamate levels, and high levels of cytoplastic calcium that intensify rigid cell walls, which creates unresponsive cell receptors. Many age-related mitochondrial dysfunctions amplify and accelerate neurodegenerative and heart disorders. Thus, both carnitines are vital to organs that need a lot of energy that depend on fat burning—for example the heart and brain.

Both L-carnitine and acetyl-L-carnitine improve function of the cells lining the blood vessels (endothelial cells) and thus lower blood pressure and help prevent heart attacks and strokes. They also help prevent arrhythmias.

If taken after a stroke, acetyl-L-carnitine can protect brain cells and reduce damage by decreasing brain glutamate levels around the stroke area. It assists the antioxidant process by increasing glutathione levels (a powerful antioxidant). It also improves glucose uptake, lowers blood sugar levels, and aids diabetics by improving insulin resistance.

Acetyl-L-carnitine will increase free radicals due to increased mitochondrial energy production, so always take it with alpha lipoic acid (another powerful antioxidant). Acetyl-L-carnitine and alpha lipoic acid can repair mitochondria and restore energy levels—*well functioning mitochondria are very important to a healthy body and delays the aging process.* However, do not take this with anti-depressants as the result could be over stimulation of brain cells. Also, do not take this supplement if you have had seizures, as it could potentiate them.

Acetyl-L-carnitine aids in mild to moderate erectile dysfunction, as does pycnogenol, hesperidin, and L-arginine (the precursor to nitric oxide, which dilates blood vessels to improve blood flow). These are better than testosterone replacement therapy, which can cause an enlarged prostate and even cancer.

CLA (conjugated linoleic acid) is the conjugated form of the omega-6 fat, linoleic acid. Conjugation refers to a mixture of geometric variations of linoleic acid from two double bonds at various positions in the fatty acid 18-carbon chain.

CLA is a healthy version of the fat that reduces cancer risk and growth of most cancers, and lowers LDL (better than a statin drug, with fewer side effects). It lowers triglycerides and reduces inflammation by reducing vascular endothelial cell wall damage, so it is protective from atherosclerosis (prevents LDL and omega-6 fats from oxidizing). It improves brain function and protects from strokes and injury. CLA helps reduce harmful visceral fat and may help in losing cutaneous fat while gaining muscle mass.

Refrigerate all oils to prevent oxidation. Take with mixed tocopherol and tocotrienols (vitamin E), which protect CLA from oxidation. Pregnant moms and those breast feeding, should not take CLA as it may increase risk of migraines in the baby, later in life after birth.

CoQ10 See ubiquinol for a full description.

Curcumin is an organic soluble plant bioflavonoid extracted from the turmeric spice, a common spice in Indian curry food. It is difficult for the body to absorb unless dissolved in extra-virgin olive oil, or other fats, to make it more bioavailable. Once absorbed it is a powerful antioxidant and anti-inflammatory agent. It will calm an inflammatory cytokine storm.

Curcumin easily passes through the blood-brain barrier to protect the brain from inflammation by suppressing the COX-2 inflammation-promoting enzyme. It reverses atherosclerosis and decreases oxidation of LDL cholesterol. Curcumin binds free iron, reduces brain toxicity of mercury and aluminum, and protects from glutamate over-activation of the microglia that would lead to production of beta amyloid plaques in the brain (the accumulation of which leads to Alzheimer's).

Curcumin is a very powerful anti-cancer agent. It inhibits cancer stem cell formation and prevents angiogenesis. It promotes the killing of cancer cells but has no harmful effect on normal cells.

On top of all that, there is still more good news: curcumin increases mitochondrial energy, stimulates wound healing and DNA repair, improves insulin resistance in diabetics, deters autoimmune disorders by improving immune function, protects the liver and leaky gut syndrome, reduces radiation damage from mammograms, CT, and PET scans, thins blood, and helps prevent post-stroke inflammation.

This, and quercetin, are good supplements to take before surgery to prevent post-surgical inflammation and induce healing.

DHA (docosahexaenoic acid) is one component of fish, or omega-3, oil. The other is EPA, or eicosapentaenoic acid. EPA will suppress the immune system, does not help control diabetes, and allows hemorrhaging—clearly not the better component of the two. For this reason, we want to find a supplement that maximizes DHA and minimizes EPA.

DHA protects and nurtures the brain, especially in fetal development. The brain is 60 percent fat and DHA is co-soluble, which promotes greater benefit. It decreases glutamate excitotoxicity, like magnesium, and modulates the electrical synaptic conduction.

It also mitigates the effects of strokes on patients by decreasing brain inflammation and inhibiting the microglia response. Thus, it's best to give stroke victims DHA immediately after diagnosis of a stroke.

DHA protects the heart-preventing arrhythmias, improves blood flow, promotes muscle repair, and maintains healthy blood vessels by decreasing the inflammation within them. It also helps diabetics by decreasing inflammation, while calming inflammatory cytokine storms to aid the immune system.

DHA decreases visceral fat by increasing resistance of fat cells to insulin so that the fat is not stored within the fat cells—thus it decreases the need for fat cells. It also inhibits aging by protecting the DNA in the cells.

Flaxseed oil comes from the seed of the Flax plant. Fifty-five percent of the oil is alpha linolenic acid. It is one of the two essential fatty acids not synthesized in the human body, so it must be acquired through diet. The other essential fatty acid obtained from food is linoleic acid (contrasted with linolenic acid). Alpha linolenic acid is a polyunsaturated omega-3 fat used in cooking, similar to rapeseed (canola) and soybean, but is much healthier as it is not derived by GMO plants (rapeseed) and does not contain glutamate (in soybeans).

Alpha linolenic acid from flaxseed is similar to gamma linolenic acid from Borage oil and has many medicinal benefits for the body. It will decrease hypertension, reduce atherosclerosis, decrease risk for melanoma, reduce depression, helps prevent liver disease, decreases cholesterol blood levels, and decreases risk for prostate cancer. It is also synthesized into DHA (a form of omega-3 fish oil), which has many more useful benefits as noted above.

A Harvard study in 2009 found that omega-3 deficiencies account for 72,000 to 96,000 deaths per year due to lack of intake of the essential fatty acids. The remedy is supplementation, available in liquid form or softgels. The flaxseed oil needs protection from light, oxygen, and heat to prevent its breakdown; therefore, maintain it in a dark, airtight container and refrigerate.

Ginkgo Biloba is a natural blood thinner that increases brain blood flow to protect against hypoxia (low blood oxygen) and mitigates the effects of stroke from its anti-coagulant properties. It's a good blood thinner and should not be combined with prescription blood thinners (Warfarin, Coumadin) as the effects can potentiate and lead to uncontrollable bleeding. It would be wise to stop taking gingko biloba two weeks before surgery.

It also improves insulin sensitivity, reduces liver damage from fats by reducing oxidation of fats (and thereby reduces atherosclerosis), reduces obesity and abnormal blood fatty acids, and improves memory and learning.

Glutathione is one of the antioxidant network heavy hitters. It performs its antioxidant role in the cell nucleus and cytoplasmic mitochondria, which protects from free radicals. Glutathione levels decrease with age and with eating foods high in glutamate. Rejuvenation occurs by increasing levels of vitamin C, NAC (N-acetyl cysteine), and magnesium—compounds that increase this nutrient's biological synthesis.

High glutathione levels help protect the body from getting cancer and decreases cancer tumor growth. It also reduces metastasis through preventing natural stem cells from turning into cancer stem cells. This is due to the neutralizing of free radicals, which would otherwise cause DNA damage in normal stem cells. Please note, stem cells are discussed in detail in the Cancer section of Chapter Seven.

Glutathione is extremely important for detoxification in the body by liver cells—and thus slows aging. However, acetaminophen (Tylenol) destroys glutathione in the liver and causes irreparable liver damage. Acetaminophen is the most common cause for acute liver failure in the US and associated with hundreds of deaths per year, even at recommended doses. Acetaminophen depletes cellular glutathione, which then renders these cells susceptible to infections, toxins, and disease. Impaired liver detoxification from low glutathione levels can predispose a person to massive liver failure and the inability to fight infection and toxins.

Do not give kids Tylenol for fever or viruses, as it will not help the fever and will weaken the liver's ability to fight the infection.

Glutathione also chelates mercury, aluminum, and excess iron, and then removes them from the body.

Grape Seed Extract is a bioflavonoid in the anthocyanins group. It is a powerful antioxidant and anti-inflammatory, which helps people with Parkinson's by protecting the brain from glutamate. It will also stabilize atherosclerotic plaques in blood vessels so part of the plaque will not break off and create a blockage (embolus) downstream.

Grape seed extract promotes heart health, prevents angiogenesis in cancer tumors, and decreases the absorption of iron by the body.

Green Tea Extract (EGCG) is the extract of the bioflavonoid group catechins, with the name epigallocatechin gallate (EGCG). It reduces atherosclerosis risk by inhibiting the free radical and lipid peroxidation effects of iron in blood vessels, strengthens blood vessel walls, and reduces hypertension. It reduces visceral fat by inhibiting sugar and fat absorption into the adipose tissue. EGCG corrects blood lipoprotein levels by reducing total cholesterol, elevating HDL, and reducing triglycerides. It helps control carbohydrate metabolism and absorption by improving insulin sensitivity so more sugar absorbs into the cells. It also reduces advanced glycation end products (AGE's).

Epigallocatechin gallate is also brain protective and has anti-cancer properties—it inhibits angiogenesis.

Hawthorn is a bioflavonoid of the epicatechins group. It reduces blood pressure by dilating blood vessels, strengthening blood vessels and heart muscle for stronger contractions, and reducing heart failure and palpitations. As an antioxidant, it protects the walls of major blood vessels from inflammation of lipid peroxidation from omega-6 fats oxidation.

Hawthorn also protects the brain against stroke damage by reducing brain inflammation and shortness of breath.

Synergistic effectiveness can occur with simultaneous prescription anti-hypertensive drugs. Therefore, lower the dosage of these prescription drugs—thereby reducing their harmful side effects. Make sure to consult with your cardiologist first. The maximum dosage for Hawthorn is 1800 mg/day, which is a high threshold.

Hesperidin is a bioflavonoid group found in citrus fruits. It is an antioxidant and anti-inflammatory that decreases brain excitotoxicity while stimulating brain derived neurotrophic factor (BDNF), which repairs damaged nerves; and it protects against AGE's. In addition, it fights cancer and reduces radiation damage from mammograms, CT, and PET scans, while preventing angiogenesis and decreasing iron absorption. Furthermore, it aids diabetics by preventing increased blood fatty acids and stabilizing blood sugar.

Hesperidin increases nitric oxide, which dilates blood vessels to increase flow thus inhibiting erectile dysfunction. It doesn't increase nitric oxide levels in the brain (as seen with L-Arginine below), which can form the free radical peroxynitrite. Note: the superoxide radical combines with the nitric oxide to form peroxynitrite, a powerful free radical associated with many neurodegenerative diseases, like dementia.

Hesperidin should only be used for three to six months; any longer can cause the side effects of stomach upset and pain, diarrhea, and headaches. If any of these symptoms occur, discontinue use or reduce dosage. It also reduces clotting of blood, so be sure to stop using it two weeks before any surgery.

L-Arginine is an amino acid constituent of protein. It boosts immunity to fight infection. L-arginine also increases insulin sensitivity but can worsen reactive hypoglycemia, so use it with caution. It may also cause diarrhea and worsen gout.

L-arginine aids erectile dysfunction by increasing nitric oxide to dilate blood vessels throughout the entire body, including the brain. Elevated brain levels can lead to peroxynitrite build-up, which causes inflammation, possibly leading to dementia. Always take it with antioxidants such as alpha lipoic acid to prevent peroxynitrite-induced dementia.

L-Carnosine consists of two combined amino acids, to protect the heart and brain where concentrations of it are higher. In the heart, it decreases arrhythmias. In the brain, it is an antioxidant so it prevents neurodegenerative diseases, such as Alzheimer's and Parkinson's, by interfering with beta-amyloid production.

Through its antioxidant property, L-carnosine helps slow down aging from chronic inflammation and free radical production, which shortens lifespan. It also aids in the mitigation of cataracts.

AGE's (advanced glycation end products) result from a high sugar intake that causes a reaction between sugar and proteins that produce free radicals, which oxidize omega-6 fats to cause inflammation. Carnosine helps prevent and dissolve AGE's.

As carnosine reduces the formation of AGEs, it can reduce the development or worsening of many diseases such as diabetes, atherosclerosis, and Alzheimer's. It also inhibits the growth of cancer tumor cells. The primary source is beef and poultry, so vegetarians must supplement their diet with this nutrient.

MCT oil, or medium chain triglyceride oil, consists of medium length chains of 8 to 12 carbons. Coconut oil is a good source of this alternate energy during glucose shortages and especially for ketogenic diets to starve cancer cell growth. MCT oil increases insulin efficiency and mitochondrial function while reducing microglia activation and thus inflammation, while also protecting the brain.

Taking large quantities of MCT oil all at once can lead to stomach cramps and gastrointestinal upset. Do not take more than two to three tablespoons at any time. If you experience cramps, reduce the amount of MCT oil. Conversely, if you do not feel cramps, your body may be able to tolerate a slightly higher dosage. Your body will tell you what it will allow.

Melatonin is synthesized in the pineal gland of the brain, the center that modulates sleep and the circadian rhythm. It is a powerful antioxidant and promotes brain healing. Alzheimer's patients have very low melatonin levels, aiding inflammation and dementia.

Melatonin levels decline after age 40 and is very low by age 70. This is why the elderly have a harder time sleeping. Excitotoxins also affect the pineal gland and further decrease its production.

Melatonin also helps enzymes to repair DNA and prevent cancer in the entire body. The usual dose is 5 mg taken 30 minutes before bed. Do not drive or operate equipment after taking melatonin.

Multivitamin is a preparation of supplements and minerals in one pill, to aid and boost the diet in supplying needed nutrients. They provide various benefits to specific groups of consumers targeted to receive different formulations. Various multivitamins exist for children, men, women, and "mature age 50+", plus other designations. Multivitamins are intended to be taken once or twice a day. Because the amounts of each component are small, consumers are generally advised to take additional, specific

CHAPTER THREE | NUTRITIONAL SUPPLEMENTS

supplements and minerals to provide adequate biofunctional levels.

NAC (N-acetyl cysteine) replenishes glutathione, the powerful antioxidant. N-acetyl cysteine (NAC), glutamic acid, and glycine bond together in cells to form Glutathione. NAC is the limiting factor in the synthetic process –it is obtained from plant sources and supplementation. Do not take NAC supplements on an empty stomach as it can cause cramping and stomach pain.

NAC can interfere with some chemotherapy drugs used during active cancer treatment; For this reason it would be better to take borage oil (for the DGLA effects) and other supplements that battle all phases of cancer, rather than submitting to chemotherapeutic agents. Take NAC and other anti-inflammatory/antioxidants daily for a lifetime to prevent cancer.

Probiotics are the good gut bacteria that we want to maintain and promote in our intestines. "Pro" means "to be for, or favor," whichever word follows this prefix. In this case, the core word is "biotic," which means a living organism, such as bacteria. Therefore, probiotics means favorable bacteria. Compare this with anti-biotic, which means "against the bacteria," referring to something that kills them, such as penicillin.

Probiotics are bacteria such as Lactobacillus, Bifidobacterium, and Acidophilus. These probiotics perform vital functions. They fight the "bad" bacteria in the gut (like the harmful species of E. coli.) and aid the immune system. Beneficial intestinal bacteria also help digest and absorb food, help generate special nutrients (for example vitamin B-12), prevent food allergies, and help repair the gut lining.

The intestine and colon account for 80 percent of our immune system function and produce the all-important immunoglobulin A

(IgA), which protects the entire GI (gastrointestinal) tract lining. Probiotics help metabolize hormones and keep gut bacteria in balance to maintain a healthy immune system. In contrast, antibiotics can kill off many of the good intestinal bacteria, to the point when probiotics become necessary to counter-balance the immune system when antibiotics have been prescribed.

Probiotics, the friendly bacteria, influence the immune system regarding which foods the body will tolerate and which foods against which to develop a reaction or intolerance. This process begins shortly after birth, so for newborns, do not give antibiotics, which would kill off good bacteria and set the child up for food allergies or intolerance down the line. Probiotics may even help prevent later cancers. Antibiotics, especially given long-term, can increase greater risk of developing cancer due to the reduction of good bacteria—thus inhibiting the immune system. Healthcare providers, and from the ubiquitous requests of patients, tend to over-prescribe antibiotics—possibly another cause for the dramatic rise in cancer we see today.

Dysbiosis is the imbalance created between good versus bad intestinal bacteria. Excessive bad bacteria promote indigestion, bloating, gas, constipation and diarrhea due to fermentation of undigested carbohydrates. An imbalance of gut bacteria can also cause yeast infections, gingivitis, halitosis, bladder infections, immune deficiencies, and even colon cancer. For example, IBS (irritable bowel syndrome) results from dysbiosis due to a reduction of the healthy good gut bacteria.

Not all brands of probiotics are effective. They need to pass through the stomach—and strong stomach acids—to reach the intestines. The dose should contain at least 5 billion total organisms to insure that a significant number of good bacteria reach the intestine. Some brands require refrigeration to prolong the bacterial lifespan, while others are room temperature tolerant. I find it easier to use probiotics that do not require refrigeration, especially if I am out of town, but will refrigerate them until needed.

Aging is associated with decreased immune function and directly linked to the gut bacterial flora. A proliferation of harmful bacteria can lead to chronic inflammation, cytokine release, and eventually to cancer. In addition, probiotics are important to keep the gut bacteria in balance so that chronic gut inflammation does not affect brain inflammation and lead to chronic brain microglial stimulation and dementia.

Like the intestine, the oral cavity has good and bad bacteria. We have over 300 different oral bacteria living in our mouths! Antibacterial mouth rinses can kill off good bacteria and lead to overabundance of bad bacteria, causing halitosis and gingivitis. Oral Lactobacillus reduces these harmful bacteria and improves gingivitis and halitosis. There are mouth lozenges available to treat this. Periogard® prescribed by your dentist is an antimicrobial mouth rinse that kills specific bacteria responsible for gingivitis.

Pycnogenol is an extract from pine bark and grape seeds. A powerful antioxidant, it protects the brain from injury, strokes, and neurodegenerative diseases, and it improves memory.

Pycnogenol also protects blood vessels from lipid peroxidation, which prevents vessel leakage and venous insufficiency, while reducing varicose veins. Pycnogenol increases blood levels of Nitric Oxide (NO). Therefore, along with hesperidin and L-arginine, it can aid mild to moderate erectile dysfunction.

PQQ stands for pyrroloquinoline quinone. *The most profound feature of PQQ is the maintenance and synthesis of more mitochondria.* We have examined mitochondria; they are vital to health and preventing disease. PQQ also slows down the aging process.

PQQ aids in metabolism by creating more mitochondria. This attribute has wide-ranging effects: decreasing diabetes by promoting glucose consumption via glycolysis, inhibiting the aging process by preventing premature mitochondria damage, and obstructing cancer stem cell formation from failure of mitochondria and the resulting inflammatory response.

PQQ is also an antioxidant, which relieves oxidative stress. If taken before a stroke occurs, it will mitigate the damage. It can also reduce heart muscle damage caused by restriction of the blood supply.

Quercetin with Bromelain is a bioflavonoid found in apples, cilantro, and onions. Quercetin compliments curcumin, as both are powerful anti-inflammatory and antioxidant agents. Both are fat-soluble so dissolve them in olive oil for better absorption by the body. With quercetin, the added bromelain helps absorption as well. Bromelain is a proteolytic enzyme found in the stems of pineapples. As an anti-inflammatory, it relieves ulcerative colitis and breaks down the protein build-up seen in the visual field known as "eye floaters".

Quercetin, as an anti-inflammatory, will calm visceral fat inflammatory cytokines, prevent and reduce atherosclerotic plaque build-up, prevent heart attacks and strokes, act as an anti-coagulant that thins blood and lowers blood pressure, lessen the after effects of strokes, and improve insulin resistance.

CHAPTER THREE | NUTRITIONAL SUPPLEMENTS

As a powerful antioxidant, quercetin prevents the oxidation of LDL cholesterol, reduces AGE's, decreases excitotoxicity from microglial activation in the brain (thus protecting it from glutamate induced beta amyloid plaque), reduces free radicals and lipid peroxidation (which decreases the effects of diabetes), and reduces radiation exposure damage from diagnostic imaging.

Quercetin also fights cancer by killing cancer stem cells, preventing angiogenesis, chelating iron, increasing mitochondrial energy, stimulating the healing and repair process, and aiding chemotherapy while protecting normal cells.

Wow, Quercetin is a powerful bioflavonoid! Too bad few people know its many benefits. Quercetin and curcumin are heavy hitters and need to be on everybody's team.

Resveratrol comes from the skin of grapes, making red wine more potent for resveratrol than white wine, due to the presence of this catechin bioflavonoid. It is an antioxidant and anti-inflammatory that reduces cytokine storms, prevents angiogenesis, and reduces radiation damage to cells from mammograms, CT, and PET scans.

Resveratrol has a maximum effective dose of 500 mg per day; it can be toxic at higher doses. For the red wine enthusiasts, thankfully you cannot drink enough red wine per day to reach this maximum level.

Taurine is another diverse nutrient that is an antioxidant and anti-inflammatory agent. Along with glutathione, it protects the liver and has a major role in detoxification. It protects the heart and is essential for heart function by regulating calcium levels, preventing arrhythmias, and lowering blood pressure. It is also a major component of bile, produced in the liver and stored in the gall bladder, which aids in the digestion of fat in the small intestine. Bile has a high pH, so it neutralizes the food from the stomach.

Taurine decreases excitotoxicity and reduces LDL cholesterol from entering the blood vessel wall. If it can't enter the wall, it will not oxidize in the blood vessel; thus taurine prevents atherosclerosis from occurring in the first place. It also prevents AGE's and the resulting chronic inflammation.

Taurine can reduce blood sugar levels, so for those with reactive hypoglycemia, take it along with a meal. Otherwise, take it 30 minutes before a meal. Be careful with consuming energy drinks as some may contain 1000 to 2000 mg of taurine in each drink. This could lead to excessive bile formed, resulting in bile acid diarrhea, as the small intestine can't reabsorb the excess bile; a condition associated with microscopic colitis.

Ubiquinol is the active and more bioavailable supplement form of CoQ10. We will primarily use the term ubiquinol hereafter, but it is interchangeable with CoQ10. Ubiquinol is the fully reduced form of CoQ10 and it exists in most cells to protect us from free radicals.

Cells synthesize this nutrient; therefore, this vital antioxidant is not required in the diet. Ubiquinol is part of the antioxidant network in cells and synthesized by a 17-step process that requires seven vitamins and several minerals. This is similar to a process used to make cholesterol; and statins that lower cholesterol, will also lower ubiquinol levels. Ubiquinol is present in the mitochondria of all cells, which regulates metabolism and energy production, especially in heart muscle.

Ubiquinol is very important to proper heart function, as it

CHAPTER THREE | NUTRITIONAL SUPPLEMENTS

needs a lot of energy. Without it, the heart muscle cells would die from lack of energy and would lead to congestive heart failure. Note if you need heart surgery, pre load with Ubiquinol (and magnesium) and you will get better post-operative results.

Ubiquinol prevents oxidation of LDL cholesterol and thus prevents atherosclerosis. It also removes excess iron from cells. Iron is a major cause of free radicals and lipid peroxidation, which precipitates cancer, heart attacks, and strokes.

The antioxidant action of ubiquinol is one of the most important functions in cellular biology; it is an essential component of the mitochondrial electron transport chain to transfer electrons during the synthesis of ATP in creating chemical energy. Without ubiquinol, cells would not manufacture energy and they would die.

Ubiquinol protects the cell membranes (lipid bilayers) against lipid peroxidation and damage, while also regenerating the other antioxidants: vitamin C, vitamin E, and the alpha tocopherol component of vitamin E.

It also supplies the brain with energy and as an antioxidant to rid excitotoxins and prevent ALS (Lou Gehrig's disease), Alzheimer's, and Parkinson's disease. Ubiquinol is fat-soluble and taken in liquid form for better absorption. Remember, the brain cells and cell walls in general, are mostly lipid, so ubiquinol moves through these structures more easily to offer unique protection.

Vinpocetine is a compound synthesized from the leaf of the ground cover plant, minor periwinkle, or simply vinca. It enhances thinking, memory, and attention, by increasing levels of neurotransmitters (noradrenaline, dopamine, and acetylcholine) depleted by aging and/or neurological disorders. It raises brain adenosine levels, which protects the brain and reduces seizures.

A special property is that vinpocetine increases blood flow in the brain's arterioles, even to areas damaged by strokes. This happens without increasing blood pressure—prescription drugs cannot make this claim. It also makes RBC's more flexible so they can navigate into small capillaries and oxygenate those areas to prevent cell death, especially after a stroke, brain trauma, aging, and degenerative disorders.

It also increases brain energy but does not increase free radical production, so it reduces inflammation and excitotoxicity. It even reduces the effect of released glutamate over-activity from excitotoxicity, but allows normal glutamate receptors to function for neurotransmission. Most seizures result from excitotoxicity due to inflammation leading to over-activation of glutamate receptors—thus, vinpocetine can reduce seizures and help epilepsy patients.

Vinpocetine works by blocking sodium channels in the cell wall layer in brain and heart cells, and thus lowers intracellular calcium levels. This prevents cellular malfunction by various calcium processes, which would cause cell death. It protects the heart and brain via the mitochondria in the cells. As an antioxidant and anti-inflammatory, it could play a part in preventing and treating cancer.

Giving vinpocetine directly after a stroke can protect stroke victims from damage to the brain, especially the hippocampus (the memory/learning center). Vinpocetine can also help people with hearing loss and tinnitus due to poor circulation in the arterioles supplying the hearing neurons. Note: do not take vinpocetine with drugs that raise dopamine levels as it may cause hallucinations.

CHAPTER THREE | NUTRITIONAL SUPPLEMENTS

Aging

LET'S DIGRESS FOR a moment to discuss the physiology of aging and to learn about supplements that can delay this inevitable process. Aging is the process of living things becoming older and more frail. For our purposes, we will address human aging from the cellular level. In 1961, anatomist Leonard Hayflick determined that normal human cells divide between 40 to 60 times before the cell division stops and natural cell death occurs. **Apoptosis** is the natural, programmed death of cells after a certain number of DNA replications have occurred. Human tissue cells divide our entire life; so what makes division finally stop?

One theory is that cell death results from DNA damage to the point that self-replication is no longer possible, and cell division fails to occur. These non-divided cells will then undergo apoptosis due to cell damage. To understand how DNA damage occurs, we need to look at the structure of DNA. At the end of the DNA's genetic double helix strands are nucleic acid sequences called telomeres. Telomeres are DNA-protective end-caps that prevent the strands from unraveling and becoming damaged—much like the plastic end-caps on shoestrings.

When the DNA replicates and the cells divide, a small portion of the telomere clips off and becomes shorter. With excessive replications, the DNA telomere becomes too short to be protective, and the DNA strand is unraveled and defective to the point where cell divisions fail to occur. This is what we call aging—the widespread occurrence of older and damaged cells.

The premise behind the 2015 movie, "The Age of Adaline" was that Adaline's telomeres failed to shorten with replication, so she could undergo unlimited DNA replications with cell divisions, and thereby not age.

Another cause for normal cell telomeres to shorten, and thus reduce the number of times the DNA can replicate, is due to free radicals that cause lipid peroxidation. We have seen how this promotes chronic inflammation and results in damage; but here, it damages the telomeres and allows the DNA to unravel.

Other causes of cell damage can accelerate aging. AGE's (advance glycation end products) result from a high sugar intake that causes a reaction between sugar and proteins to oxidize omega-6 fats to produce these end products. They are free radicals that produce inflammation and damage cells, promoting aging.

Aged cells also accumulate from the progressive loss of mitochondrial function, resulting in less energy production for cells to utilize. This is especially significant in the heart and brain tissue; heart disease and dementia are serious problems among the elderly.

Mitochondrial dysfunction creates more free radicals, causing chronic inflammation and consequently leading to mitochondrial failure—thus, a detrimental cyclic downward spiral.

We have seen how inflammation is the primary cause of most diseases. What goes hand-in-hand with inflammation is mitochondrial dysfunction. Which one causes the other? Depending upon circumstances, inflammation may cause mitochondrial dysfunction, or mitochondrial dysfunction may cause inflammation. The final result is the same—disease. Therefore, it is prudent to prevent and treat both in every case, as one always leads to the other.

That which causes inflammation poisons the mitochondria, this includes industrial chemicals, pesticides, herbicides, fungicides, vaccinations, MSG, mercury, lead, cadmium, aluminum, and systemic fluoride.

As we age, our body produces more free radicals, which oxidize and destroy the cells. Also, mitochondrial energy wanes with age and more free radicals occur—at age 70 we have 10 to 15 times more free radicals than at age 35—and more corresponding inflammation.

The effects of aging are inevitable; what can we do to slow its progress? The best measures to promote longevity are having good nutrition, taking vitamin and mineral supplements, exercising, getting enough sleep, and avoiding stress, pollutants, and chemicals as best we can. This sounds overwhelming; is it even possible? The answer is yes, thankfully, and it will entail more information, provided in the following chapters.

Antioxidants neutralize caustic free radical particles and protect the telomeres from damage. The antioxidant network (Vitamin C, Vitamin E, Ubiquinol, Glutathione, and Lipoic Acid) works within the cells to reduce this oxidative stress and damage. Also important are B vitamins, acetyl-L-Carnitine, Vitamin K, magnesium, zinc, and PQQ.

Aging is associated with decreased immune function, which can lead to chronic inflammation and cytokine release. Vitamin D3 will improve immune function along with probiotics. The use of probiotics is important to keep the gut bacteria in balance so the immune system is not overburdened—thereby fending off the occurrence of chronic gut inflammation. Also beneficial to reduce inflammation is curcumin, quercetin, and DHA.

The dentist in me will tell you there is a direct link between gut health, body health, and brain health, all of which relates to gum health. So, brush and floss regularly to help maintain total body health and to slow the aging process.

References

The Holy Bible, the Book of Genesis.

http://www.heart.org/HEARTORG/Caregiver/Replenish/WhatisaServing/What-is-a-Serving_UCM_301838_Article.jsp.

Blaylock, R.L., Blaylock wellness reports, Feb 2014.

Blaylock, R.L., Blaylock wellness reports, Oct 2012.

Mohamad, S.B., et. al., Comp Biochem Physiol A Mol Integr Physiol 2002; 132: 1-8.

Yamamoto, N., et. al., Transl Oncol 2008; 1(2): 65-72.

Benthsath, A.; Rusznyak, S. T.; Szent-Györgyi, A. (1937). "Vitamin P". *Nature* 139(3512): 326–327. Bibcode:1937Natur.139R.326B. doi:10.1038/139326b0.

http://www.mensfitness.com/nutrition/what-to-eat/6-reasons-to-never-neglect-flax-seed.

http://www.globalhealingcenter.com/natural-health/the-health-benefits-of-flaxseed-oil/.

Blaylock, R.L., Blaylock wellness reports, June 2011.

CHAPTER FOUR
Exercise

Regular exercise extends life expectancy and healthy years . . . Exercise is about as effective as medications in preventing death from cardiovascular disease and diabetes. The results are even better when combined with proper nutrition.

The Benefits of Exercise

JACK LALANNE LIVED to be 96 years young. He was the epitome of a healthy life through exercise and nutrition. The Jack Lalanne Show, which aired from 1951 to 1985, showed America that exercise promotes good health. Exercise was important then and even more so today. Proper exercise is **The Fourth Secret** to develop a leaner, stronger body while avoiding cancer and other diseases. Let's look at the numerous benefits of exercise and why it is the fourth secret.

Primarily, exercise develops muscle tone and increases muscle bulk. Better muscle tone allows us to carry on everyday activities with ease and with less chance of injury. As we age this is even more critical; prevention of fractured hips due to falls would save the elderly from painful and lengthy hospital stays. Loss of muscle mass and strength is a problem with aging and causes imbalance, leading to falls and injury. Hence, exercise becomes more important for muscle tone in the elderly, but it does not have to involve rigorous weight lifting.

Secondary benefits of exercise involve stimulation of the brain's growth repair hormone, **BDNF** (<u>b</u>rain <u>d</u>erived <u>n</u>eurotrophic <u>f</u>actor) which improves brain plasticity. BDNF repairs brain damage by increasing nerve dendrites and synapses, and increases brain blood flow, especially in the hippocampus. This part of the brain is the center of memory and learning—the primary area affected by Alzheimer's patients who have low levels of BDNF.

BDNF also acts on the neurons in the brain's hypothalamus to secrete more leptin, the satiation hormone, so we are less hungry and lose weight. It reduces the risk of diabetes by diminishing insulin resistance, and that decreases blood sugar levels by promoting sugar uptake by muscle cells for metabolism. With glucose absorbed by cells and insulin levels reduced, the chronic inflammation promoters (free radicals and lipid peroxidation of omega-6 fats or glycation products) diminish, and we see a reduction or prevention of disease and cancer risk.

The brain releases endorphins after exercise, especially after anaerobic exercise from weight training. This neurotransmitter, felt after a workout, makes us feel good. It is the "runners high" that is felt during longer (anaerobic) runs.

CHAPTER FOUR | EXERCISE

Exercise also increases the level of antioxidant network enzymes, lowers blood pressure, improves lung function, strengthens immunity, slows down aging, and inhibits depression. As we can see, there are numerous benefits to exercising—unfit men are six times more likely to die from a heart attack than are fit men.

Weight resistance training exercises the muscles and strengthens the skeletal system, tendons, and ligaments. The stress placed on bones creates a healthy physiological process, whereby the bone constantly remodels itself through cells that break down bone (osteo<u>clasts</u>) and those that build up bone (osteo<u>blasts</u>). The production of excess free plasma calcium also occurs through exercise, which promotes uptake into the bones and makes them harder.

Exercise improves blood and lymph flow to tissues and organs by dilating the vessels. The deep breathing during exercise causes the release of nitric oxide, which dilates vessels and increases the flow of lymph in lymphatic vessels (especially the heart and lung); this cleanses the tissues from toxic chemical build-up.

Greater exercise intensity correlates with larger brain volume and gray matter; which corresponds to fewer signs and symptoms of Alzheimer's. On the contrary, the lack of exercise is the most powerful risk factor in predicting the odds of developing dementia. Maintaining an exercise schedule even into the golden years will keep them memorable (literally!).

Exercise causes sweating to occur, which removes toxins through the skin. Therefore, it is important to drink water before, during, and after a workout to prevent dehydration. This will facilitate metabolism and aid in the regeneration of muscle cells.

One should even consider dissolving electrolyte tablets in drinking water to replace lost minerals. Nuun® makes tasty electrolyte tablets with no added sugar that dissolve in water.

Muscle Cell Physiology/Weight Training

SARCOMERES ARE THE basic unit in muscle, which consists of long fibrous proteins that slide past each other upon muscle contraction and relaxation. A group of sarcomeres form a **myofibril**, and a group of myofibrils form a muscle cell or **myofiber** (myo is the Greek root word for muscle). The accumulation of all muscle cells forms the entire muscle. As an interesting side note, a single muscle cell may contain 100,000 sarcomeres, the fibrous proteins that facilitate its contraction.

The **sarcoplasm** surrounds the myofibrils and is similar to the cytoplasm of other tissues. It contains a large amount of stored glycogen (carbohydrate) granules—for ATP energy production to facilitate muscle sarcomere contraction—and **myoglobin**, which is a protein to bind and carry oxygen to the mitochondria for metabolism.

When we exercise, we target both the myofibril and the sarcoplasm. Each contributes to muscle bulk while burning more fat in the process. Weight resistance training causes the myofibrils to incur micro-tears that regenerate with more sarcomeres, thus resulting in greater bulk and strength. Due to these micro-tears in the sarcomeres, it is important to allow that muscle group to rest at least two days before exercising those same muscles, to let the body heal itself and create more sarcomere protein. This is critical to prevent muscle fiber scar tissue and damage.

The sarcoplasm content adapts and increases due to extended tension on the muscle (muscle fatigue); this allows for muscle expansion or bulk. Giving short rest breaks between sets of muscle group exercises further enhances the adaptive regeneration process.

Muscle creates the ability to move, maintain balance, engage in everyday activities, and do so much more. Muscle increases metabolism to burn more calories by increasing insulin sensitivity while sugar absorption by muscle cells dominates fat storage. After you exercise, metabolism continues, and carbohydrate burning occurs even at rest or while sleeping for up to 24 hours. Fitness gurus will tell you their exercise program will burn calories even while you sleep—actually, all exercises will do this. The evidence for this occurs in a higher core temperature after working out, which can even persist during sleep. Weight training also boosts growth hormone (GH); this burns fat and stimulates the production of more muscle fiber. Growth hormone, called the "anti-aging hormone," unfortunately diminishes, as we get older.

There are three types of muscle cells in the human body: cardiac, smooth, and striated. The striated, or skeletal muscle cells, are most numerous and provide the body with support and movement. The "striation" appears because when viewed through the microscope these muscle cells appear to have light and dark bands. A few familiar examples of these muscles are biceps, triceps, quadriceps, and trapezius.

Cardiac muscle appears only in the heart, while smooth muscle occurs in tissues and organs that require involuntary control to perform its function. For the purpose of exercise and weight training, only skeletal muscles will be examined in detail.

The skeletal muscles can be divided further into slow-twitch (Type I) or fast-twitch (Type II). Slow-twitch, or "red" muscle fibers have many capillaries that give it the red color. It also has abundant mitochondria and myoglobin. This thinly sized muscle will sustain a slow contraction for long periods. It is resistant to fatigue, as it has more oxygen provided to the mitochondria; but it has low contractile force. These tonic fibers turn on (undergo contraction) in variable fiber amounts, as needed, to provide and maintain continual postural support and stability for the body. They function in various standing and sitting positions; thus, these slow-twitch muscles envelop the core or mid-section of the body.

The **aerobic** (with oxygen) metabolism in the slow-twitch muscle uses fats and carbohydrates to fuel the process. Marathon runners have generally adapted to more slow-twitch muscles to sustain the long distance run. Weight training that develops these muscles utilizes lighter weights and maintains 25 or more repetitions per set.

Fast-twitch muscles contract more quickly and with more force, but also fatigue rapidly. These muscles are phasic; they either produce a contraction or are relaxed, with no in-between condition. These fibers have two sub-groups, fast-twitch Type IIa and fast-twitch Type IIb.

The fast-twitch Type IIa muscle falls into more of an intermediate group as the moderate-sized muscle is red in color and has numerous mitochondria and abundant myoglobin, but contracts somewhat quickly. That is, it produces a moderate degree of contractile force and is somewhat resistant to fatigue. This muscle is adapted to perform high-intensity anaerobic, activities that are of intermediate length—less than 30 minutes—such as swimming. It primarily utilizes glycolysis (anaerobic—without oxygen) metabolism for the ATP energy source, but can use the citric acid cycle (aerobic—with oxygen). Weight training for fast-twitch Type IIa muscle involves lifting intermediate weights with 10 to 25 repetitions per set.

Fast-twitch Type IIb muscle consists of thick sized "white" muscle as they have low mitochondria and myoglobin concentrations. They fatigue easily but produce a quick and powerful contraction. This fiber supports short anaerobic activities that last less than a minute, such as sprinting and weight lifting. The primary energy source is glycogen through the ATP process, which delivers a lot of energy but regenerates slowly. Weight training for fast-twitch Type IIb fibers involves lifting less than 10 repetitions per set and with heavier weights.

Skeletal muscles are comprised of a mixture of different fiber types, depending on the purpose for that muscle. Muscles can adapt and generate more of one fiber depending on need. For example, core postural muscles are predominantly Type I fibers because they sustain contractions, do not need to produce a lot of power, and are very resistant to fatigue. In addition, when a muscle contracts, only the needed fibers will contract. If a weak contraction is required, only the Type I muscle fibers will contract. If a strong contraction is called for that requires a lot of power, the Type IIa and IIb fibers will be activated along with the Type I fibers; but the Type IIa and IIb fibers will activate only after the Type I fibers.

Since there are different fiber types (I, IIa, and IIb), we need to exercise and train each muscle differently, according to their function and fiber composition. The Type I fibers are more static in nature, that is, they create a long-term contraction. We must compliment this feature by performing static training to build this muscle. For example, *the core trunk muscles that provide stability and balance benefit from isometric or static exercises.* These

HEALTHY BODY, HAPPY LIFE

involve activation of muscle fibers that do not rely on movement by contraction or extension of the fibers. An example is the plank exercise, where the body remains in motionless tension. This exercise, and many others, will be described in Chapter Six.

To illustrate this point let me tell you about a personal experience. Soon after graduating from dental school, I noticed I could not sleep for more than five hours before developing severe lower back pain that woke me up and prevented me from getting back to sleep. This was probably due to elongation of the spine during sleep and the stretching of the core muscles—my abdominal and back muscles were out of balance from not getting any exercise. During the day, the problem was relieved: the force of gravity on my spine compressed the discs, and the muscles were therefore not over-stretched, so I did not experience pain. However, I could not go on living like this; I was simply not getting enough sleep.

In an attempt to remedy my lower back pain, I played basketball weekly with some friends to get some exercise to help correct the imbalance. It helped a little with the back pain, but not enough. Then I started going to a gym and did abdominal exercises (crunches). Although this helped, it still did not provide 100 percent relief. Soon after that, core exercises like the plank and isometrics were discovered to be the answer, and now I have no lower back pain and can sleep a normal seven to eight hours. The key here is that the muscle fibers need exercise according to their type; without it, one gets only minimal results, and in my circumstance, the pain remained.

Skeletal muscles that allow movement of limbs are dynamic in nature and require training through motion to mimic natural bodily movement. These engage the Type II fibers while the weight training exercises involve muscle contraction and extension. Examples are biceps curls, squats, bench presses, etc. With these muscle groups, we want to use dynamic weight resistance training that includes performing 10 repetitions through motion.

Strength training should build muscle without putting extreme stress on the joints. It is better to work out with moderate weights to prevent any possible damage. The process relies on high muscle fatigue with short rests between sets.

Free weights are better than machines and universal gyms as they force one to use opposing muscle groups to balance the weight through a motion. Weight machines generally have one directed pathway that removes the stabilizing requirement needed from counter-balancing muscle groups. You get a better complete workout when free weights are used. Free weights also promote functional body movements and the corresponding strength training that will assist the body in undertaking normal, everyday activities.

Knowing which fiber we are trying to target can greatly assist in toning and adding bulk to the specific muscle. This will also aid in training muscles that assist our normal, everyday life activities, which will help to prevent falls and injuries; that is especially important, as we get older.

We can use muscle cell physiology to our advantage during weight training by incorporating two factors to add more bulk to fast-twitch Type II muscle fibers. First, it is only through micro-tears of the muscle fibers that we get deposition of new protein formation in the sarcomeres.

To promote more of these micro-tears, we need to contract the muscle through a full range of motion. Thus, it is important to acquire full extension of the muscle before a weight-resisted contraction occurs. This promotes controlled micro-tears along the entire muscle that will later heal to form more bulk.

For example, doing abdominal crunches on the floor does not allow a full range of contraction of stomach muscles. It is better to use a workout ball to do crunches—but remember to arch your back fully to stretch the abdominal muscles before doing the crunch. This will better develop the muscle group over a full range of motion and thereby deliver more bulk.

The second factor we can utilize to maximize our workout is the mechanics of the weight resistance training. This includes the number of repetitions, the number of sets, and the timing between them. That is, we need to focus on the fast-twitch Type IIb fibers and the sarcoplasm. This will produce the greatest bulk. Let's see how to achieve this.

For any strength training exercise, start with a free weight that you can lift about 15 times before the muscle fatigues and you can't do any more. This will be your starting weight for that exercise. Remember, it is always better to start lighter and get your system down before proceeding to the heavier limits of your capability. Do 10 repetitions with that starting weight, then rest that muscle group for 40 seconds. Perform another set, then rest for 40 seconds again. Do four complete sets, but on the last set do as many as you can while maintaining proper form. If you can only perform a few repetitions on the last set, consider using slightly lighter weights the next time. If you can do more than 10, consider next using slightly heavier weights. Keep a record of the weights used to monitor your progress.

During Type II fiber weight training, we are aiming to achieve total muscle fatigue, or failure, on the last set, for the biggest gains. To gain the most benefit out of weight resistance training, it is best to utilize equal periods for weight-training repetitions and the rest between sets. In addition, the ideal number of sets is four. This creates a balance between myofibril and sarcoplasm stimulation to provide the best muscle generation. *If one performs more sets with lighter weights, the sarcoplasmic process is favored; and if one does heavier weights with fewer sets, the myofibril process prevails.* Remember, in life we strive for balance.

It is important to use moderate weights for these strength-training exercises. This prevents excessive stress on bones, tendons, and ligaments; a benefit appreciated in our older years. It may be impressive to your gym friends that you can lift the heaviest weight possible . . . But are we trying to obtain the envy or admiration of our peers at the expense of our body, or are we trying to promote a healthy body?

The speed by which one performs strength training is also important. Contraction of a muscle group should be around one second, while the extension or muscle lengthening phase should be three seconds. The contraction pulls the sarcomeres across each other, and the extension stretches and pulls them to create the micro-tears. Thus, the lengthening phase has the most impact on myofibril production. This timing, results in a 40-second set—ten repetitions at four seconds per repetition (4 X 10= 40 seconds). When coupled with the 40-second rest phase, we get the equal balance between tension and rest, to create equal amounts of myofibrils and sarcoplasm.

It is important to realize where the contraction or shortening of the muscle occurs. For example, the biceps curl will have a one-second contraction with the upward movement, while the relaxation phase occurs while lowering the weight. The squat will have the one-second contraction of the quadriceps when raising the body up and the relaxation period is lowering the body downward. This is important so we can remember to use proper timing and breathing techniques with contraction and extension of various muscle groups.

Breathing

BECAUSE BREATHING IS perhaps one of the most fundamental and vital actions that we as humans perform on a consistent basis—literally, every second of our daily lives!—it deserves particular attention.

The normal adult has an average respiratory rate of 16 to 20 breaths per minute. The purpose of breathing is to expel carbon dioxide (the by-product of our constant cellular metabolism via the citric acid cycle) and exchange it for oxygen, used to create cellular levels of NADH for cell metabolism. This process in the lungs of swapping oxygen for carbon dioxide allows cellular mitochondria to produce the ATP energy molecule. However, this process requires maintaining a balance. Improper breathing can result in many catastrophic events. Let's see why.

The carbon dioxide levels in our body help regulate blood pH. Hyperventilation, in which we breathe in and out too fast, blows off excessive amounts of carbon dioxide. This results in dizziness, headache, tingling lips, weakness, and even fainting or seizures. We have all experienced a mild form of this when blowing up too many balloons at a birthday party and feeling lightheaded.

The loss of too much carbon dioxide can cause the bronchiole

CHAPTER FOUR | EXERCISE

smooth muscles to constrict and induce an asthma-like response that results in feeling we can't breathe. The normal reaction is to breathe harder and deeper. However, this only makes matters worse as less oxygen is actually absorbed and more carbon dioxide expelled. Moreover, this causes further blood vessel restriction, which can reduce the blood flow to the heart and possibly lead to cardiac arrest. The treatment is simple. Grab a bag (or cup your hands around your mouth if no bag is available) and breathe in and out into the bag until you feel better. This builds the blood carbon dioxide levels back up into a balanced state.

Many people may not even know they hyperventilate or breathe incorrectly; and this can have negative effects during exercise. Here are some signs that will alert you to the fact that you may be breathing incorrectly: mouth breathing, frequent sighing, needing to take large breaths prior to speaking, upper chest breathing (not utilizing the diaphragm), erratic/labored breathing when at rest, sleep apnea, and constant sinus congestion or having a relentless runny nose.

There are ways to overcome these improper breathing habits. Be consciously aware if you are mouth breathing, or not utilizing your diaphragm to breathe more deeply; then retrain yourself to get into the habit of breathing through your nose and using the diaphragm to breathe correctly. That is, you should consciously take slow deep breaths down lower into the stomach area. Use the diaphragm to breathe, more so than expanding just the upper chest. Deep breathing with the diaphragm pulls more air deeper into the lungs and creates a more efficient exchange of carbon dioxide for oxygen.

Proper exercise reduces sighing, taking large breaths before speaking, and erratic and/or labored breathing. Nose breathing is instrumental in preventing congestion and a runny nose. For those of you with sleep issues, treating sleep apnea with an oral sleep aid or a C-PAP machine helps keep the airway open.

Learning to breathe correctly can improve your fitness and health by increasing oxygenation to all muscles, tissues, and organs. This will lower blood pressure and improve your endurance, mental focus, and brain health in addition to reducing stress and anxiety.

It is very important to breathe through your nose—this is something that cannot be stressed enough. Breathing through the nose profoundly affects the body, in many ways. The nose humidifies the air so the lungs do not dry out and thereby become inflamed. Remember that chronic inflammation is a cause of cancer. The nose also warms the air before it enters the lungs. This is especially critical in frigid weather, which can potentially freeze and damage the lung alveoli (the area where oxygen and carbon dioxide exchange takes place).

Breathe in deeply and steadily with your diaphragm to fill the lungs to obtain full oxygen saturation. The oxygen then transports to the various tissues for cellular metabolism. With proper oxygen levels available to supply mitochondria, cells perform at their peak ability, and the risk of oxygen deprivation leading to cancer is minimal. Recent studies have shown that hyperbaric oxygen treatment shows promise in treating cancer.

Nose breathing during exercise will help with endurance, energy levels, and performance. Even more beneficial, the nose has nitric oxide gas that enters the lungs. We have seen before, when describing the benefits of the supplements (L-arginine, hesperidin, acetyl-L-carnitine, and pycnogenol), an increase in nitric oxide production helps dilates blood vessels. Nitric oxide in the lungs not only dilates the bronchioles and blood vessels, but it has antimicrobial properties that help to kill germs. Thus, it serves to help prevent a chronic runny nose and congestion.

Breathing through the nose helps maintain a steady breathing volume, which alleviates hyperventilation and the associated imbalance of blood pH. The nasal passages are not as large as the throat, so the tidal volume of air in and out is slower, more steady, and longer in duration.

Breathing during weight training and exercise should be through the nose for the reasons stated above. Many trainers advocate breathing out of the mouth during a contraction of a muscle group, and breathing in through the nose, during extension. The understanding is that there is less resistance with mouth breathing, and it is easier. Yet this does not allow for the benefit to the body of increased nitric oxide. So, as much as possible, breathe in and out through your nose. However, it is better as trainers say, to breathe out during a contraction of the muscle as this prevents strain on the diaphragm and core muscles—but the lesson here is to do it all through your nose.

With the resistant weight training technique, breathe out during the one-second contraction of the muscle group, and breathe in deeply to fill the bottom of your lungs during the three-second extension. This combines the best breathing technique with the best mechanics for optimal muscle mass gain.

Stretching

STRETCHING THE MUSCLE groups before weight training and physical activity is critical to prevent injury. Numerous books and internet sources fully discuss this topic. Because it is important, but not the main focus of this book, the reader is encouraged to research other material on this subject.

Extreme Exercise

LACK OF EXERCISE leads to a host of ailments; but does extreme exercise cause harm as well? When we think about extreme exercise, the marathon runner comes to mind. They train for hours without stopping. The downfall with this practice is that it depletes the body of glucose (which gets used up first), followed by glycogen (or stored glucose), then fat; and finally, since there is no other energy source, protein breaks down and metabolizes as fuel. This is why marathon runners do not have large muscles; they have Type I and Type IIa muscles to go the distance. In contrast, the sprinter will have the large Type IIb muscles because their training requires short bursts of explosive force.

Is extreme training unhealthy in the end? It can be, so take proper steps to counteract the pitfalls. The increased metabolism associated with long-term intense training increases free radicals and lipid peroxidation of fats that promotes chronic inflammation. We have seen how this leads to diabetes, cardiovascular disease, and cancer. It is important to take antioxidants as they rid the body of these excess free radicals and prevent inflammation.

Also harmful to the body, extreme exercise depletes magnesium and ubiquinol levels. Magnesium helps prevent arrhythmias, and ubiquinol aids the mitochondria with energy production in the heart. Therefore, the depletion of either can create a serious problem. Have you ever heard in the news about the healthy high school or college aged basketball player who suddenly collapsed on the court and died from sudden cardiac arrest? They probably suffered from very low magnesium and/or ubiquinol levels, leading to heart failure. The sad thing, this is preventable by making sure of proper supplementation and nutrition. If you engage in rigorous training, get your magnesium and ubiquinol levels checked, and supplement them as needed.

Aerobic Exercise Training

AEROBIC EXERCISE, SUCH as a treadmill workout, helps oxygenate tissues, which prevents cancer. This is because the cancer tumor cells prefer an anaerobic environment (without oxygen) and get their energy from glycolysis (anaerobic metabolism).

However, this is a double-edged sword in that circulating oxygen can become a free radical that can last for hours after exercise. Therefore, it is best to maintain proper antioxidant intake to prevent the free radical damage from the oxygen free radicals.

Physical activity requires increased levels of oxygen. Therefore, it is best not to exercise by roadways, as cars and trucks emit large quantities of carbon monoxide, leading to oxygen starvation in the brain. This would result in inflammation and stimulation of the microglia—and associated neurological problems.

Long-term aerobic exercise proves to be minimally beneficial for the heart and the burning of calories. New studies have shown that a different approach is better than hours on the elliptical machine, which only develop the Type I and Type IIa muscle fibers. We need a better way to stimulate the Type IIb fibers while also increasing oxygenation, improving blood flow, and stimulating the body to produce healthy proteins and hormones.

High-Intensity Interval Training (HIIT)

HIGH-INTENSITY INTERVAL training became popular around 2010. HIIT involves interval training that alternates short, intense anaerobic exercise with low-intensity recovery periods. The exercise and recovery periods can vary, but one effective regimen involves intense exercise for 30 seconds followed by a low-intensity recovery period of 90 seconds. That one cycle lasts two minutes; perform eight cycles for a total of 16 minutes. With a two-minute warm-up and two-minute cool-down, plus the 16-minute exercise regimen, HIIT requires only 20 minutes total. That is a vast improvement over the 30 to 60 minutes for traditional treadmill aerobic exercise—and even with a busy lifestyle, one can easily find 20 minutes in front of the TV to complete the regimen. And the good news, HIIT also promotes all three muscle fiber types.

One can use a variety of activities for the short intense exercise phase. It can be on the elliptical machine (my preference) where you choose the resistance level and angle of incline for the intense phase, then slow down at a lower incline for 90 seconds. Alternatively, you can run in place while moving your arms, even with light dumbbells, for 30 seconds, then walking for 90 seconds. If a swimming pool is available, use your favorite swim stroke. If you are close to a track, running for 30 seconds while walking for 90 seconds also works. Be creative—there are many possibilities!

HIIT is a form of cardiovascular exercise that improves glucose metabolism by lowering insulin resistance and increases fat burning by enhancing muscle fat oxidation. It also enhances athletic capacity and conditioning, as well as increasing levels of growth hormone. The aerobic benefits of HIIT have been studied and determined to deliver the same amount of biochemical changes and endurance as those who trained four times longer with traditional treadmill aerobic training. HIIT also increases the resting metabolic rate for the following 24 hours, due to increased oxygen consumption. Thus, one burns more glucose and fat well after the workout.

So let us sum this up. HIIT requires less time, it improves metabolism and fat burning well after the fact and it improves athletic performance and conditioning. I like this!!! The only thing HIIT will not do is improve muscle bulk. That is the purpose of weight-resistance training; and we can actually employ intense-interval training for that as well. We have talked about this when discussing fast-twitch Type IIb fibers—using moderate weights during a set for 40 seconds, with 40 seconds of rest in between sets. We will call this **HIST**, for **high-intensity strength training.**

Both HIIT and HIST provide the best of all beneficial features of exercise and in a fraction of the time. To understand evolution and the physiological necessity of such exercise, we need to look back again at the lifestyle and physical needs of ancient humans for survival.

Just like other predatory mammals, such as lions, the human bodies were designed for highly intense, but short-burst activities. During evolution, the need to hunt food involved short sprints to chase wild game (HIIT); and when we caught the animal, a wrestling match ensued to subdue the wild beast (HIST). Mankind evolved to function in accordance with that need, and we can employ this physiology to promote better workouts and health.

Let us also examine the cellular and chemical benefits of HIIT and HIST. High-intensity interval and strength training promote the release of myokines produced by muscle fibers. Myokines are cell-signaling proteins that are anti-inflammatory and thus combat metabolic syndrome (high blood pressure, obesity, diabetes, and high blood levels of omega-6 fats) and cancer.

Myokines are in the class of cytokines. As you may recall, cytokines produced in visceral fat are inflammatory cytokines, such as TNF-alpha (tumor necrosis factor alpha) and IL-1 (interleukin-1). Muscle cells act as an endocrine system, producing myokines that are anti-inflammatory, which counter the effects of inflammatory cytokines. Myokines are extremely beneficial in that they reduce metabolic syndrome factors by increasing insulin sensitivity, and increase glucose utilization in muscles. They also promote the burning of the fat in muscles and fat liberation from adipose cells, which inhibits the release of visceral fat inflammatory cytokines. Myokines also reduce body fat generation, regardless of caloric intake. *More proof that exercise is extremely important for overall health.*

The body likes and needs balance, and we are healthier when we have that equilibrium. There must also be a balance between myokines and inflammatory cytokines or the inflammatory cytokines will dominate and cause disease. Myokines from exercise cannot counteract a poor diet of refined sugar (especially HFCS), grains, trans fats and processed foods; the inflammatory cytokines will win. It is easier to eat less of these bad foods than exercise them away. You will see how this is possible in Chapter six.

The best workout routines include both HIIT and HIST. However, the body needs recovery time. It is important to give your muscle groups at least two days to recuperate before pushing them again. You will know if you are pushing your body too hard: constant body fatigue is a sign of overdoing the exercise program. You should feel slightly fatigued after a workout, but soon recover and feel great due to the release of endorphins. They are the natural pleasure neurotransmitter in the brain.

High-intensity strength training requires at least two days per week to target all muscles; and high-intensity interval training should be done two to three times per week. Personally, I like to break up the HIST workout days by doing HIIT on the off days.

Strength training is more important as we age to prevent falls that can be life threatening, improve circulation, and release myokines to reduce inflammation and prevent cancer. It also lowers risk of diabetes and metabolic syndrome, and it is good for you psychologically as you look and feel better.

Utilizing intermittent fasting and HIIT/HIST together can reap huge benefits for weight loss. Both of these lifestyle changes shift the body into fat burning mode for the primary fuel source. And it is important to have a nutritious diet with healthy omega-3 fats (avocados, DHA, MCT oil, coconut oil, olive oil, flaxseed oil, and raw nuts), and cut down on fructose (eat low fructose fruits), glucose, and especially HFCS (in soda pop). Eat good protein such as free-range chicken or grass-fed, hormone-free beef. Even better, you can eat all the vegetables you want—the amazing thing about eating less sugar is that fresh organic vegetables will taste so much better, and you will actually crave more of them.

The Importance of Protein after a Workout

WHAT AND WHEN you eat after exercise training is critical. A common misconception is that muscles develop from lifting weights. This is not true. During the workout, we have effectively torn the muscle fibers—at this point, no fiber synthesizes to the muscle to provide more bulk. You build muscle fiber and bulk during the recovery phase, which can take hours to a couple of days afterward. This is where diet is critical.

Since muscle consists of protein, we need to consume protein in order to repair and build muscle tissue; but not just any protein will do. Protein consumption must also occur within the first hour after training to gain the most benefit. Many protein products claim to build bigger, better, faster muscles. The first thing to examine is the protein label: remember the label-reading example of that popular protein drink? Make sure that what you ingest is full of good, nutritious ingredients. We will look at my recipe for a refreshing protein drink later, in Chapter Six. However, for now, we will look at some protein basics.

For the body to build muscle during the recovery phase process, it needs amino acids—the protein building blocks of muscle fibers. The **branched-chain amino acids** (BCAA) are very important in this regard to repair and build more muscle. The muscle building branched chain essential amino acids are leucine, isoleucine, and valine. When you read the product label, make sure the protein has as much of these three as possible. They are anabolic, which means the muscle cells use them to build muscle fiber and thus bulk.

Let's digress a moment to learn the meaning and nature of **"anabolic"** and **"catabolic."** Metabolism is the complex set of biochemical processes that occur in the cells of the body to sustain life. Metabolism consists of two opposing features; catabolic is the biochemical processes that break down molecules into smaller ones while anabolic is the biochemical processes that build larger molecules from smaller ones.

Catabolic metabolism involves breaking down nutrients into smaller molecules, while generating energy molecules to perform other specific body functions. For example, glucose breaks down into carbon dioxide and water and releases ATP (adenosine triphosphate) energy, which the muscles then harness for contraction. It also creates smaller building-block molecules (carbon dioxide and water), which the body will either excrete or later use to create larger, more complex molecules during an anabolic process.

Anabolic metabolism involves building new, more complex molecules, to synthesize body components like the phospholipid cell walls, or muscle fiber. These anabolic processes are also very important for the body to repair damaged tissue.

There are better forms of protein that contain higher levels of the BCAA's. They must also be digested and readily absorbed to build muscle. The best proteins, in descending order, are whey protein, whole eggs, chicken, beef, and fish. Whey protein is a vital adjunct to post-workout nutrition that increases cell repair and recovery; it is the recommended source of protein. Whey protein comes in two forms, isolate and concentrate. The concentrate form is 30 to 89 percent protein, while the isolate is above 90 percent protein. We want to use the isolate form with the higher concentration of protein.

Diet and exercise are two very important factors in maintaining health and a long life. Aging causes muscle strength to decrease plus a reduction in muscle size. Protein is important for muscle growth and even maintenance of the muscle mass we already have. Nevertheless, there must be a balance of protein consumption.

The caveat here, though, is to realize that an all-protein diet is not healthy; too much protein can be a problem as well. Excess protein can lead to the conversion of protein into sugar and then into fat. This can lead to increased visceral fat, with the corresponding increase in inflammatory cytokines and inflammation. In addition, sugar fuels cancer growth.

Many body builders subject themselves to excessive protein diets, which can cause kidney damage. If the diet continues for extended periods, kidney failure can result from the removal of excess nitrogen waste products in the blood during protein metabolism. Body builders also have an overall shorter lifespan, increased risk for heart and brain damage of the hippocampus (the learning/memory center), and cancer. Switching to a healthy protein, low caloric diet reduces heart disease, cancer, diabetes, and neurodegenerative diseases.

The high concentration of the amino acid glutamine, found in popular protein supplements, can also be detrimental. Intracellular processes convert it into glutamic acid, and the salt form, glutamate. Even though it is within the cells, high concentrations of glutamate can exit cells and have adverse effects on the brain and cancer receptors.

Glutamine is a conditionally essential amino acid that plays a part in protein synthesis and regulation of acid-base balance (pH) in the kidneys via ammonia (more specifically nitrogen). It is a source of cellular energy, and donates nitrogen for many anabolic processes. Glutamine also donates a carbon during the citric acid cycle, and is the non-toxic transporter of ammonia in blood circulation. Thus, it is important in a balanced diet, but the excitotoxic nature of glutamine in high brain concentrations can result in unwanted, over-activation of the brain microglia, resulting in dementia. The good news is that exercise helps deplete the blood of harmful glutamate for use in muscle energy production. Nevertheless, as in all metabolic processes, moderation is the key.

References

Erickson K.I., et al., Hippocampus 2009; 19: 1030-1039.

Blaylock, R.L., Blaylock wellness reports, Sept 2010.

Mattson M.P., et al., Trends Neuroscience 2004; 27: 589-594.

Wilburta Q. Lindh; Marilyn Pooler Acleod SA. Human skeletal muscle fiber type classifications. Phys Ther. 2001;81(11):1810-6; Carol Tamparo; Barbara M. Dahl (9 March 2009). Delmar's Comprehensive Medical Assisting: Administrative and Clinical Competencies. Cengage Learning. p.573. ISBN 978-1-4354-1914 8.

British Journal Clinical Pharmacology. May; 29(5): p.519-524.

Perry, Christopher G.R.; Heigenhauser, George J.F.; Bonen, Arend; Spriet, Lawrence L. (2008). "High-intensity aerobic interval training increased fat and carbohydrate metabolic capacities in human skeletal muscle". Applied Physiology, Nutrition, and Metabolism 33(6): 1112-23. PMID 19088769.

Gibala, M. J.; Little, J. P.; Van Essen, M.; Wilkin, G. P.; Burgomaster, K. A.; Safdar, A.; Raha, S.; Tarnopolsky, M. A. (2006). "Short-term sprint interval versus traditional endurance training: Similar initial adaptations in human skeletal muscle and exercise performance". *The Journal of Physiology* 575 (3): 901–11. PMID 16825308.

Sowers, Strakie. "A Primer On Branched Chain Amino Acids" (PDF). Huntington College of Health Sciences. Retrieved 22 March 2011.

Shimomura Y, Murakami T, Naoya Nakai N, Nagasaki M, Harris RA (2004). "Exercise Promotes BCAA Catabolism: Effects of BCAA Supplementation on Skeletal Muscle during Exercise". *J. Nutr.* 134 (6): 1583S–1587S.

Livestrong, October 21, 2013.

WebMD, April 22, 2002

CHAPTER FIVE
More Health Hazards

Boosting health hasn't been tried yet in modern medicine.

WE HAVE ALREADY looked at the health hazards of statin drugs, vaccines, and GMO's. They are unsafe and their avoidance recommended. Nevertheless, they are actually only the tip of the iceberg; there are more harmful practices to scrutinize and avoid.

The Cell Phone

THE FIRST MOBILE phone call aired in 1973. From that early stage until now, the use of cell phones has exploded to over 7 billion worldwide by 2014. Cell phone technology improved immensely over this period, allowing people to communicate anywhere in the world by voice, pictures, text, and through the transfer of data.

With improvements in lithium batteries, the power of the phone has also magnified. *However, what are the hazards of holding such power so close to the body, and more importantly, to the intricate network of nerves in the human brain?*

Cell phones use microwaves to receive and transmit digital information. By comparison, the microwave oven cooks food by the use of microwaves. Just what are these electromagnetic radiation waves and what are the ones in cell phones doing to our bodies? Do they "cook" human tissue? In 2011, the World Health Organization classified the cell phone as "possibly carcinogenic to humans."

A meta-analysis study conducted in 2009 by V. Khurana concluded that cell phone use for at least 10 years, showed twice the risk of developing a brain tumor on the same side of the head as the side of cell phone use. Remember that Phil's lesion, desmoplastic melanoma, was above the left ear—his preferred ear for listening on the cell phone. Another study reported a 40 percent increased risk of a cancerous brain tumor (glioma) when the user talked an average of 30 minutes per day for over 10 years.

On February 22, 2011, CNN aired a report that discussed the effects of cell phones on the brain. They reported that Dr. Volkow performed a study and determined that the level of brain activity was associated with the amount of glucose metabolized to create brain fuel. They also noted that the area of the brain closest to the antenna of the cell phone had significantly more brain activity and metabolized more glucose than when the cell phone was off. *Thus, the microwaves are stimulating the brain into over activity.*

Dr. Ronald Herberman, the former Director of the University of Pittsburgh Cancer Institute, stated the following:

> *"We know that increased glucose also occurs with infections and other inflammatory processes, and leads to the production of potentially damaging reactive oxygen radicals that can alter the ways that cells and genes work. This important finding should stimulate many biologists to perform in-depth studies to determine the consequences of such changes in nerve cells or other bodily cells in the region of the radiation. We need to develop a better understanding of how radiofrequency radiation might contribute to increased risk for brain tumors as well as other alterations in brain functions."*

One can conclude that chronic exposure by cell phone microwaves can lead to excitotoxicity, over-activation of the microglia, and ultimately brain glioma or other diseases. A frightening question arises about the effects to the developing brains of children who use cell phones. This is critical considering the brain continues to grow and develop until the age of 26.

The good news is that there are preventive measures we can use to reduce the exposure to cell phone microwaves:

1) Keep the antenna as far away from your head as possible. The best solution is to use an earpiece that conducts sound through an air tube, much like a stethoscope. If this is not feasible, use a wired head set. There are still electromagnetic fields involved with these products, but the reduction of the intense radiation is worth it. What people do not consider is that Bluetooth technology still places microwaves very close to the brain.

2) Another method is to keep the cell phone away from your head at least six inches by placing the phone on speakerphone mode. Microwave amplitude (intensity)

is inversely proportional to the square of the distance away from the source. This means that if you double the distance the antenna is away from your head, the intensity of the microwave is one-quarter of the original energy; and if you make it three times the distance, the energy is one-ninth as strong.

2) Keep the cell phone away from your body in general. Findings show a link between men who carry the cell phone in their pocket with decreased fertility. Women have seen increased rates of breast cancer on the side where they tuck the phone in their bra. A purse is a better place to carry the phone; and better yet, place it farther away whenever possible.

3) Use texting to communicate. This method is not as fast as talking directly, but it keeps the phone away from your brain and reduces cancer risk.

4) Use a conventional alarm clock. Using the phone for an alarm clock or placing it under your pillow subjects you to unwanted microwaves, even if no calls are made. Studies show that having the phone anywhere in the bedroom will disrupt a person's sleep; and loss of sleep creates other unwanted health concerns.

5) Use a special cell phone case that can block and reduce radiation by up to two-thirds.

6) Restrict the use of cell phones by children. They are not toys and shouldn't be treated as one.

7) Cordless phones emit radiation too. Use the speakerphone when possible, and keep it away from your body as much as possible.

8) Use the landline when possible.

9) Limit the use of other wireless devices such as a keyboard, mouse, laptop, and/or router.

10) Do not reside within 600 feet of cell phone towers. They emit concentrated levels of microwaves.

The Microwave Oven

THE FIRST RESIDENTIAL countertop microwave oven was manufactured and available for public use in 1967. Its development was based on World War II radar technology and utilized microwaves to heat food quickly in warzones. However, are these timesaving food warmers safe?

Microwave ovens rely on waves of electrical and magnetic energy to vibrate water molecules rapidly, at millions of cycles per second. The friction produced is what heats up the food. The reason why ceramic plates and bowls do not get warm is that they have no water in the material. If the containers do get warm, it is due to heat conduction from the food itself.

So what does this violent, high-friction heat do to food? Heating food by stovetop methods creates some nutrient loss in food, but the "microwave effect" is even worse.

In 1995, a scientist named Kakita demonstrated that microwaves can severely fragment and destroy viral DNA. Other studies have found that numerous food nutrients change chemically when microwaved and become carcinogenic, especially the amino acids in proteins.

Various studies show the following:

1) Microwaved broccoli lost 97 percent of its antioxidants, compared to steamed broccoli, which lost 11 percent.

2) Microwaved asparagus caused a reduction in vitamin C.

3) Microwaving garlic for 60 seconds destroys the active ingredient that fights cancer.

4) Six minutes of microwaving inactivates 30 to 40 percent of B12 in milk.

5) Microwaves cause more protein to "unfold" than conventional heating—thus destroying the properties of the protein by altering amino acids.

6) Breast milk degrades more by microwaving than other warming methods.

7) It is also best to microwave items in ceramic dishes; plastic can leach out BPA (bisphenol A) which is absorbed by food. BPA is an estrogen-like compound that can alter hormone and cause cancer.

Make sure the microwave oven is functioning properly and the door closes tight to prevent leakage of microwaves. Even with these precautions, standing just one foot away exposes one to 400 milliGauss of radiation—4 milliGauss has been linked to leukemia. In addition, a study published in Medical News Today in February 2014, by Dr. Havas of Trent University found that microwave radiation frequency affects the heart at levels well below federal safety guidelines.

People can even experience microwave sickness if exposed to

high levels of microwave radiation. Some symptoms include headaches, vision problems (even cataracts), sleep problems, depression and irritability, suppressed immune system, nausea, and the inability to think clearly.

To reduce exposure to actual microwaves and the effects of microwaved foods, there are alternative measures to having a microwave oven. The main requirement is to plan ahead so foods can be thawed and heated by the stovetop, regular oven, or even a convection oven. However, not all foods need reheating—I enjoy cold pizza the day after going to the local pizzeria.

Aluminum

ALUMINUM IS THE third most abundant element on earth and the most abundant metal. It occurs naturally in many different minerals.

Drugs, vaccines, food, and household products bombard us with aluminum. Drugs such as analgesics, antacids, and anti-diarrheals contain aluminum. We have discussed vaccines, so now we will look at food and household products. The number one food source for aluminum is soy, which is also high in glutamate. This toxic combination is readily absorbed into the bloodstream, which stimulates the microglial immune response.

Sea salt contains aluminum, as well as black tea. Citric acid found in fruits will increase absorption of aluminum, so do not put lemon wedges in your black tea, as this will increase blood levels of aluminum and increase excitotoxicity in the brain.

The cooking ingredient Alum contains aluminum, found in pickling juice and baking powder. We also find aluminum in coffee creamers, processed foods, and caking agents. Through lists investigated on the Internet, we can learn about the harmful levels of aluminum present in various foods.

Aluminum exists naturally in the air, water, and soil. We ingest seven to nine mg (milligrams) of aluminum per day from our environment, but the good thing is that our body only absorbs around 1 percent. Household products like antiperspirants, cosmetics, shampoo, and sunscreen can all contain this excitotoxic mineral—it is important to read product labels.

Aluminum is also made into "aluminum foil" for wrapping around and cooking food. Refrain from this practice—the aluminum will leach out and contaminate the food. Avoid aluminum soda pop cans and buy bottles instead.

Cookware can also be a concern. Pots and pans made of iron and copper will react with vitamin C found in many foods and turn the ascorbate into a free radical—dehydroascorbate. The iron itself is a known free radical when unbound in the blood, and Teflon used in non-stick pans is carcinogenic. Aluminum utensils are not a good choice either. The only choice for safe cookware is stainless steel. They may be a little more expensive to purchase, but your health is worth the price.

We have already discussed the excitotoxic effects of aluminum in detail (see Chapter Two), which causes Alzheimer's in the hippocampus (memory/learning center in the brain), but there is a recent study that illustrates just how lethal aluminum can be.

A case study from Keele University in England, reported in the Journal of Medical Case Reports (February 10, 2104), showed a direct link between aluminum and Alzheimer's. The report describes how a 66-year-old man working in the aluminum industry for eight years, continually breathed in aluminum dust and developed early onset Alzheimer's from accumulated and elevated levels of aluminum in the brain. This link between aluminum and Alzheimer's is not surprising given the increasing number of people who are acquiring this horrible condition and, too often, at a younger age.

Now the question becomes how we purge our bodies of this toxic element. As with all other conditions, prevention is far better than requiring a cure. Try to avoid aluminum contamination in the first place; so please read product labels. Since absorbing aluminum is practically impossible to prevent due to its ubiquitous presence, the next best step is to detoxify the body of existing aluminum. Chelating agents are molecules that will bind with these minerals and facilitate their removal from the body.

Melatonin is an antioxidant that also chelates, or binds aluminum. It readily crosses the blood-brain barrier to bind and remove this toxic metal. Curcumin is also very useful as it binds aluminum and decreases the beta-amyloid plaque seen in the brains of Alzheimer's patients, which may help to improve memory. This is in addition to curcumin's excellent anti-inflammatory and antioxidant properties.

Glutathione is the body's main detoxifying antioxidant. To boost glutathione levels we have seen that supplementation with NAC (N-Acetyl-Cysteine) is very important. Also helpful is vitamin D3, exercise, and maintaining dietary sulfur levels. Once again, this is proof that proper diet and supplementation are critical to a balanced and healthy life.

Sleep Disorders

SLEEP IS AN altered state of consciousness that involves anabolic processes to build up the muscular, skeletal, nervous, and immune systems. In humans, the sleep regimen is usually at night, normally for seven to nine hours.

The sleep requirements for healthy rejuvenation do not have to be continuous hours, naps can also provide anabolic renewal—siestas are a normal part of many cultures.

Sleep deprivation promotes many ailments and these disorders caused by insomnia, sleep apnea, and snoring result in oxygen deficiency.

Insomnia is the inability to fall asleep or stay asleep as long as desired. The cause is from stimulants (caffeine or drugs), pain, stress (increased cortisol levels), restless leg syndrome, or poor sleep environments.

To rule out poor sleep environments eliminate noise, do not eat food or drink alcohol three hours before bed, do not engage your mind in stimulating activities right before bed (television or computer), keep the room dark, remove all sources of microwaves (cell phones, cordless phones, routers, etc.), and have the temperature turned down a few degrees. Restless leg syndrome improves by supplementing with L-Tyrosine, magnesium, and alpha lipoic Acid.

Insomnia is more common in the elderly, women, and people under stress. Increased visceral fat in the elderly produces insomnia-causing cytokines that cause inflammation, which affects the circadian clock rhythm, the 24-hour sleep pattern cycle influenced by periods of light and dark. The elderly also produce less melatonin in the pineal gland, which regulates and aids the sleep pattern. Supplementation with 5 mg melatonin will reverse this shortage.

Women tend to experience more insomnia due to lower hormone levels of progesterone during menstrual cycles and lower estrogen during the post-menopausal stage. Hormone replacement therapy with estriol can decrease hot flashes and regulate the circadian rhythm. Estriol is a natural hormone in women. Note, the use of Premarin, or estradiol, can increase the risk for breast cancer.

Stress causes harm to the body in many ways and affects sleep through over-production of cortisol. This awakening hormone is responsible for making the brain alert in times of stress. It is a defense mechanism, along with the fight-or-flight response. People with insomnia produce more cortisol at night, and the brain is too alert to fall asleep. Many natural supplements are available to aid with stress, depression, and anxiety, such as melatonin, among others.

Sleep apnea is a condition that involves pauses in breathing due to the tongue dropping back and collapsing the airway preventing the movement of vital air; this can last from several seconds to minutes. These apneic episodes may occur many times per hour during sleep, depriving the body of much needed oxygen that can impair internal organ function and potentiate other health problems. There is an increased risk of high blood pressure, stroke, heart disease, arrhythmias, cognitive decline (Alzheimer's), and diabetes. Sleep apnea can also cause cancer due to **hypoxia** (lack of oxygen in the tissues/organs) which activates cell-signaling molecules that stimulate inflammation and allow for cancer development, growth, and spread. It is very important to keep the body well oxygenated. We can assist this task while awake by taking 10 deep breaths per hour. This is another reason exercise is good for us; it forces deep oxygenated breathing.

Carotid bodies are natural chemoreceptors attached to the sympathetic nervous system, located in the branching area of the carotid arteries in the neck. They regulate blood pressure and breathing by detecting changes in PO_2 (the partial pressure of oxygen dissolved in the blood), PCO_2 (the partial pressure of carbon dioxide in the blood), pH (the acidity of blood), and temperature. If an oxygen deficiency occurs, carotid bodies stimulate the sympathetic nerves to increase blood pressure by constricting arteries and increasing the breathing rate, by sending an impulse to the brain. Chronic over stimulation leads to enlarged heart, arrhythmias, cold hands/feet, kidney damage, high blood pressure, and anxiety—all of which can lead to heart failure. Inflammatory cytokines from visceral fat also react with the carotid bodies and trigger sympathetic overdrive leading to the previously mentioned problems.

Sleep apnea is dangerous; it is a chronic condition causing hypoxia, and then inflammation. Chronic heart failure can result in further hypoxia and drive inflammation. Glutamate also stimulates the sympathetic nervous system into overdrive—thus, diet is very important: avoid MSG, omega-6 fats, sugar (especially HFCS), sulfites, nitrites, and high glycemic foods. Hypoglycemia (from reactive hypoglycemia) can send the body into panic mode and trigger the sympathetic system into overdrive, in an attempt to increase blood sugar levels. In diabetics, this chronic condition can cause the overdrive to increase risk for heart disease, atherosclerosis, strokes, and hypertension.

CHAPTER FIVE | MORE HEALTH HAZARDS

When carbon dioxide builds up in the blood stream from lack of proper breathing at night, the brain wakes the person up in order to resume breathing and restore oxygen levels. The repeated waking does not allow for deep REM sleep, leads to fatigue and sleepiness during the day—and a common consequence is falling asleep while driving, with potentially tragic outcomes.

Those afflicted with sleep apnea rarely know they suffer from this problem—unless they awaken from sleep due to the loud noise they create themselves upon gasping after the apneic episode. Usually the spouse or sleeping partner notices the disrupted breathing and listens to hear if their beloved is still alive or dying as they gasp for air. The experience can be quite alarming!

There are common risk factors associated with sleep apnea, some of which can be remedied. Apnea is more prevalent in men (53 percent affected) than women (26 percent affected), in those who are over 40, and in those who are overweight. People with enlarged tonsils or tongues and a neck size greater than 16 inches are at higher risk. This is why during physical exams physicians started asking about neck size, usually of their male patients. A larger neck, coupled with certain anatomical structures, can block normal respiration. Other factors are alcohol consumption that relaxes the throat muscles and constricts the airway; and smoking, which promotes apneic episodes three times more likely than in non-smokers.

There are varied treatments that range from a change in lifestyle habits, to mechanical devices, to surgery. Unfortunately, we cannot do anything about our gender or age, but we can lose weight, avoid alcohol (especially before bed), and quit smoking, all of which can produce positive changes in preventing sleep apnea.

Mechanical devices, such as the CPAP (continuous positive airway pressure) for severe sleep apnea, and oral appliances for mild to moderate sleep apnea, can also prove beneficial. The severity and type of sleep apnea can be determined from a sleep study. Sleep study physicians prescribe patients with the CPAP machine, while dentists prescribe and place the oral appliances.

As a dentist who happens to snore and exhibit mild sleep apnea, I have seen the process from start to finish. The sleep study itself was an interesting (?) experience. I went to the sleep clinic where the technician put wire-leads all over my body and connected them to a monitor—then they watch you . . . As if you could actually sleep without turning over and pulling out the leads, causing the machine to alert the technician to come in and re-connect them.

If you have a sleep study done, have them prescribe a sleep medicine so you can actually get to sleep; or do the home sleep study, which has far less wires, and no strange technician coming into your bedroom to scare you.

After diagnosis with just mild sleep apnea, the physician did not recommend the CPAP machine. That was good because I am sure I would not be able to sleep with a mask on my face connected to a machine that makes some noise during an otherwise quiet night.

The next option was an oral device that advances the lower jaw forward to open the airway and prevent sleep apnea. With this apparatus, you have a plastic retainer on the upper and lower teeth, with a sliding connector between them, to force the mandible (lower jaw) forward. The problem with this situation is two-fold. First, it displaces the cartilage disc within the jaw joint, so with the appliance removed in the morning, there is a required period of

CHAPTER FIVE | MORE HEALTH HAZARDS

muscle relaxation, before the teeth can bite fully together again. Second, the muscles and tissues in the mouth and throat can adapt, requiring appliance adjustments to move the mandible even more forward to prevent sleep apnea. Long-term manipulation of this very complex joint is not a good thing.

Another oral appliance is one that fits on just the lower teeth and has a tailpiece to force the tongue in a down and forward position. This too opens the airway; somewhat like the plastic airway placed in a patient by paramedics during CPR. This approach takes time to grow accustom and was difficult for me to get to sleep—plus it made me salivate . . . A lot.

Further research led me to adhere to a few principles, which prevented my sleep apnea without having to use a cumbersome mouth appliance. A side benefit for this method is that it also decreases snoring. I had a special foam-sleeping wedge made that was six inches tall, by two feet wide and two feet long. I put this under my pillows to elevate my torso and alleviate the collapse of my airway from gravity. It is also important to sleep on either side, where the gravitational pull is not as great on the throat tissues. Do not sleep on your back where again, gravity will collapse the airway. This method seemed to work best as there was no appliance to adapt to and my snoring /sleep apnea stopped—also my bruised ribs finally healed from where my wife elbowed me to stop my snoring, so she could sleep. A good but expensive alternative to the wedge pillow is an adjustable bed where the angle and elevation of the head changes to suit your personal needs.

Snoring is often associated with sleep apnea, but not always, and caused by a constriction in the airway of the nose or throat. Vibrations due to air turbulence cause the noise, which is proportional to the force of air movement and the amount of constriction.

According to the American Academy of Otolaryngology, 45 percent of adults snore on occasion and 25 percent snore routinely. As with sleep apnea, men snore more than women and it's more prevalent in those overweight. It also gets worse with age as the throat tissues sag and restrict airflow. Snoring can reduce oxygenation of tissues, as with sleep apnea, and affect organ systems.

Prevention of snoring can be aided by sleeping on your side (not on your back), elevating your head, reducing your weight, using nasal strips to reduce the nose restriction, avoiding alcohol, and performing throat and tongue exercises to prevent sagging muscles and tissues. One good exercise is to start with your teeth together, then simultaneously open wide and take in a large breath of air through your mouth while trying to fully enlarge the airway; then close, and breathe out your nose. Do 10 repetitions daily to tone the muscles and tissues.

Prolonged Sitting

INCREDIBLY, SITTING TOO long and too often can affect your health. Our Garden of Eden ancestors did not have the luxury of chairs and sofas or automobiles. They had to walk to their destination and stand when they got there, or sit on the cold hard ground. Today, we are accustomed to sitting on comfortable furniture and traveling in "style."

The average person spends nine to ten hours sitting each day; this is in addition to time sleeping. At work, we spend 60 percent

CHAPTER FIVE | MORE HEALTH HAZARDS

of our time sitting. There is also a correlation: if you are sedentary at work, you will likely be sedentary at home. So be more active at work and at home. Get up and move about for 10 minutes each hour. Walk during the lunch hour—it is great exercise and a nice change of scenery to break up the workday.

So, what has this inactive lifestyle done to our well-being? Prolonged sitting affects many organ systems: the heart, brain, muscles, pancreas, colon, digestion, and even posture.

Excessive sitting slows blood flow and allows the build-up of fatty acids, triglycerides, and cholesterol to clog the arteries of the heart. We have seen where this causes inflammation due to free radical peroxidation of these fats, which cause atherosclerosis and heart disease. Prolonged sitting also affects the pancreas; there is a 90 percent increased chance of developing type II diabetes.

Low blood flow to the brain from a sedentary lifestyle supplies less oxygen to the brain and deprives mitochondria of proper metabolism. This sets off the microglia, causing prolonged inflammation, which can then lead to dementia and even cancer. When muscles do not get enough oxygen, they do not burn glucose stores, which results in fat storage and obesity, not to mention weak and atrophied muscles. In addition, postural strain on the vertebrae, cause lower back pain. Forty percent of people who have lower back pain spend many hours each day sitting, which does not allow vertebral discs to move and absorb enough blood and nutrients. The risk of herniated disks is also greater.

This affects digestion as well. Compression of the abdomen after a meal slows digestion that can cause cramping, bloating, constipation and even dysbiosis (imbalance of the intestinal bacteria). This can result in inflammatory bowel disease (IBD) or even colon cancer (increased risk by 30 percent).

Studies show prolonged sitting reduces lifespan. Adults who sit for six hours per day will reduce their lifespan by five years. This is associated with obesity and all of the ill-health effects that relate to metabolic syndrome. Reducing the average time of sitting to less than three hours per day may increase a person's life expectancy by two years. The mere act of standing—and better yet, walking—activates the core muscles and the large leg muscles. This drives glucose into muscle tissue for metabolism and depletes glucose, while decreasing insulin resistance, risk for diabetes, obesity, inflammation, and cancer.

People evolved to be active and to move. Unfortunately, more than half of the people in the United States do not engage in vigorous physical activity for more than ten minutes per week; and sit excessively. HIIT and HIST can be the cure to this problem, but you can start by just getting up and moving around more. There are many fitness bands and apps available to track steps, calories, and even heart rate; many will even congratulate you when you reach a predetermined goal of steps, or calories burned.

Here are some suggestions for becoming more active. Instead of driving the ATV or riding the lawnmower to the mailbox, walk. Instead of driving to the local grocery store, walk—this will also save on gas and wear-and-tear on the vehicle. If the store is too far to walk, park the car further from the entrance at the opposite end of the parking lot (this may save on door dings and scratches). If you are in a building and need to go up or down a few flights of stairs, walk—it will probably be faster than waiting for the elevator anyway. For those who sit a lot at work, you can use a stand-up adjustable desk. This desktop adjusts up or down to your height; allowing you to avoid the ailments associated with prolonged sitting. The possibilities are endless!

Food Allergies/Intolerances/Sensitivity

FOOD NOURISHES THE body, but some foods can elicit an unwanted response. Adverse reactions to food can be either an allergic reaction or intolerance. Food allergies can be life threatening, while intolerances cause unpleasant responses by the body.

The allergic reaction to certain foods involves an immune response that can range from mild to severe. Mild reactions generally manifest as a rash, itchiness, hives, vomiting, diarrhea, and swelling of the tongue. Severe reactions can result in breathing problems, low blood pressure, anaphylactic shock, and even death. The response can be immediate, from within minutes to as long as several hours after eating the **allergen** (a substance that causes an allergic reaction. The most common foods that people are allergic to are cow's milk, eggs, peanuts, shellfish, soy, and wheat.

The immune response by the body involves immunoglobulin E (IgE) which binds to the protein allergen in the food and stimulates mast cells to release histamine and other cell-mediated cytokines. Next, a full-blown immune response occurs, which can be local (swelling of the mouth and tongue) or systemic (a reaction of the whole body). The symptoms dissipate with anti-histamine and/or adrenaline via epiPen® (epinephrine administered in a single dose cartridge). Nevertheless, in the case of breathing difficulty, seek immediate healthcare intervention.

Testing for food allergies, based on a skin prick test, involves blood tests for IgE-specific food antibodies. Another method is a food challenge where the patient eats a particular food to determine if a reaction results. This can be potentially dangerous, so perform it only in a healthcare setting. Generally speaking, most people suffering from food allergies already know, or have a good indication of, the foods to which they are allergic—unless it is their first reaction. Thus, the best treatment is to avoid those foods causing an allergic response. However, with food processes that prepare many different foods in the same manufacturing plant, total avoidance may be difficult.

Food *intolerances* differ from food *allergies* in that they usually involve a delayed body reaction in one or more organ systems. They are not life threatening, but it can be difficult to ascertain which foods cause the intolerance. Symptoms appear from as early as 30 minutes after ingestion to as long as three days later, thus making diagnosis more difficult.

The causative agent of the intolerance is varied. It is usually a reaction to organic chemical components, which are either natural or artificial, and can be food additives, preservatives (sulfites), flavoring, and food dyes. It can be the lack of a digestive enzyme such as lactase in those people with lactose intolerance, where they cannot digest milk products.

On the other hand, it can be associated with the autoimmune disorder, called Celiac disease, whereby the body reacts to gliadin, a protein component found in the gluten of wheat products. These are the two most notorious food intolerances.

The presence of symptoms varies according to the cause and can manifest in one or more places. On the skin, one can find a rash, hives, or eczema. In the respiratory tract, you may see nasal congestion, infection of the sinus, phlegm that produces a cough, and asthma. The most noted area that produces symptoms is the gastrointestinal tract. Here, one may find mouth ulcers, nausea, gas, cramping, diarrhea, and/or constipation.

To determine which foods cause sensitivity, one can have an ELISA test for the IgG-mediated immune response to particular foods. The ELISA test (enzyme-linked immunosorbent assay) looks for the presence of different food antigens in blood that elicit the IgG antibody response. Each food yields a value assessed within a certain range. The values are scored as follows:

> A score of zero (value 0 to 0.1999) means no sensitivity.
> A score of one (value 0.200 to 0.299) signifies mild sensitivity.
> A score of two (value 0.300 to 0.399) depicts moderate sensitivity to that food.
> A score or three (value 0.400 and higher) represents those foods which show extreme sensitivity.

There can be several hundred foods analyzed and a score given to each one. Based on these findings, elimination testing will determine if the person is truly sensitive to that certain food.

With *elimination testing*, the foods that scored a one, two, or three from above are eliminated from the diet for eight to twelve weeks—which is how long it takes to clear the residues from the body. Then the lowest valued, number "one" scored food is reintroduced into the diet and tested for a response by the body. If a negative symptom from eating that food shows up, it is recorded and that food is eliminated from the diet. If a food provides no response from the body, then it becomes part of the permanent diet again. The next higher number "one" valued food is then re-introduced and evaluated. This process continues to test the remaining number "one" scored foods. Then the number "two" scored foods are tested, followed by the number "three" scored foods, and so on. This is a slow process but an effective one for ruling out offending foods.

Note that there is controversy as to whether or not the ELISA test is valid. The argument against having the test done is due to the high incidence rate of false positives. Even if there is a presence of IgG antibodies to specific foods, this does not equate to those foods causing sensitivities or devastating immune reactions. It may be that those were the foods eaten recently or most often. Therefore, it is important to verify the ELISA blood test for food sensitivities with elimination testing methods to rule out those suspect foods.

There is yet another method to determine food sensitivities at home, and the good news is that it is free. This process incorporates biofeedback, whereby the body detects a stress response after eating a sensitivity-causing food. Arthur Coca, M.D. developed the Coca Pulse Test for food sensitivities, and his book is available free on the internet. The theory behind the test is simple: if you eat a food that causes sensitivity, there will be a corresponding increase in pulse rate. The procedure starts by recording your baseline heart rate, and then requires you to eat a food to determine if the pulse increases, stays the same, or perhaps even decreases.

A modified version, called the LNT Coca Pulse Test, is also used. LNT stands for lingual-neural testing and relies on the communication pathway between the tongue and the central nervous system. When we taste food, neural messages are sent throughout the body; if food sensitivity is detected, the pulse rate will increase. Here, you test (taste) one food at a time, and measure your pulse. To take your own pulse, place the first two fingers of your hand alongside your windpipe and feel the carotid artery's pulse. You can also check your pulse on the inside of the wrist.

To perform this test, take a baseline measure of your pulse rate

CHAPTER FIVE | MORE HEALTH HAZARDS

for 60 seconds at least one hour after eating or drinking anything (except water). Make sure you are in a relaxed frame of mind and body, and be sure that you have been sitting, which ensures having a constant, steady heart rate. Place the test food in your mouth for 30 seconds; you may chew, but do not swallow it. With the food still in your mouth, retake your pulse rate for 60 seconds. Then record the food and result. Spit out the food, and rinse multiple times with clean water. If your pulse increases by six or more beats per minute, avoid that food: it created a stress reaction and tested positive. If you test positive for food sensitivity, stop that session; it could taint the results of subsequent food testing. If no increase in pulse occurs, test another food, and record the result. Do this for all suspect foods—but not more than five at any given test session. Note that to test eggs, the yolk and egg white must be tested separately, as there are usually less positive reactions to the yolk. Make sure you have everything you need to complete the testing for that session: once you sit down, do not get up since standing can increase your heart rate and give a false positive. Lastly, if you test positive for a food that consists of many ingredients (e.g. pizza) isolate each component food and test them separately.

Food sensitivities and some allergies can heal and dissipate over time from changing to a healthier diet and lifestyle. Leaky gut syndrome is the process in which the intestinal wall has pores through which undigested food proteins enter the bloodstream and trigger an immune response. A healthy diet and fiber can correct the leaky gut syndrome and eliminate this sensitivity. Even eliminating a problem food temporarily for a few months can convert that food back into a non-sensitive food. Therefore, one should re-test foods to see if they no longer create a reaction—re-test every three months to determine if the food still causes sensitivity.

Drugs/Alcohol/Smoking

IT IS COMMON knowledge that taking recreational drugs, consuming alcohol, and smoking cigarettes are poor health choices. There is a plethora of information on each of these subjects that will not be covered here. The reader is encouraged to seek information from the internet, other books, and healthcare providers.

Cessation of these activities is certainly beneficial to the body and indicates a wise decision in favor of good health. Just remember, "You cannot miss what you do not know." These habits are personal choices and as such are optional. If you do not use them, you will not become addicted, and you consequently cannot miss the effects about which you previously knew nothing.

References

"WHO: Cell phone use can increase possible cancer risk". CNN. 31 May 2011. Retrieved 31 May 2011.

Khurana, VG; Teo C; Kundi M; Hardell L; Carlberg M (2009). "Cell phones and brain tumors: A review including the long term epidemiologic data". *Surgical Neurology* 72 (3): 205–214. doi:10.1016/j.surneu.2009.01.019. PMID 19328536.

"World Health Organization: Cell Phones May Cause Cancer". Business Insider. Retrieved 31 May 2011.

Kakita Y, Kashige N, Murata K, Kuroiwa A, Funatsu M and Watanabe K. "Inactivation of Lactobacillus bacteriophage PL-1 by microwave irradiation", 1995.

Vallejo F, Tomas-Barberan F A, and Garcia-Viguera C.

CHAPTER FIVE | MORE HEALTH HAZARDS

"Phenoliccompound contents in edible parts of broccoli inflorescences after domestic cooking" Kidmose U and Kaack K. Acta Agriculturae Scandinavica B 1999:49(2):110-117.

Song K and Milner J A. "The influence of heating on the anticancer properties of garlic," Journal of Nutrition 2001;131(3S):1054S-57S.

Watanabe F, Takenaka S, Abe K, Tamura Y, and Nakano Y. J. Agric. Food Chem. Feb 26 1998;46(4):1433-1436.

George D F, Bilek M, and McKenzie D R. "Non-thermal effects in the microwave induced unfolding of proteins observed by chaperone binding," 2008 May;29(4):324-30. doi:10.1002/bem.20382.

www.ncbi.nlm.nih.gov/pubmed/18240290.

Quan R (et al) "Effects of microwave radiation on anti-infective factors in human milk," Pediatrics 89(4 part I):667-669.

Havas M. "DECT phone affects the heart!" Medical News Today February 13, 2014.

Neuro Endocrinology Letters 2005 Oct;26(5):609-16.

"Several Sleep Disorders Reflect Gender Differences". *Psychiatric News* 42 (8): 40. 2007.

Teran-Perez, G.; Arana-Lechuga, Y.; Esqueda-Leon, E.; Santana-Miranda, R.; Rojas-Zamorano, J.A.; Velazquez Moctezuma (2012). "Steroid Hormones and Sleep Regulation". *Mini reviews in medicinal chemistry* 12 (11): 1040– 8.doi:10.2174/138955712802762167. PMID 23092405.

"Sleep Apnea Health Center". An undated WebMD informational.

Yan-fang S, Yu-ping W (August 2009). "Sleep-disordered breathing: impact on functional outcome of ischemic stroke patients". *Sleep Medicine* 10 (7): 717–9.doi:10.1016/j.sleep.2008.08.006. PMID 19168390.

BMJ January 21, 2015.

BMJ Open 2012;2:e000828.

Feb 2014 "Food allergy: Epidemiology, pathogenesis, diagnosis, and treatment.". *J Allergy Clin Immunol* 133 (2): 291–307; quiz 308. doi:10.1016/j.jaci.2013.11.020. PMID 24388012.

CHAPTER SIX
The Garden Of Eden Lifestyle; A Practical Paradigm Shift

Preventative health makes a lot of sense, but it doesn't make Big Pharma a lot of money.

You are what you eat.

"Insanity is doing the same thing over and over again, and expecting a different result."
~Albert Einstein

THIS CHAPTER ASSEMBLES all the details of previous chapters to create the ultimate structure for the paradigm lifestyle change. *The Garden of Eden Lifestyle approach will be illustrated so you can easily follow the steps to develop a leaner body while preventing cancer and promoting good overall health—allowing the opportunity to pursue a happier life.*

Our culture is in desperate need of a change. Eighty percent of Americans will die from one of the top 10 causes of death (listed in descending order): heart disease, cancer, COPD (chronic obstructive pulmonary disease), stroke, accidents, Alzheimer's, diabetes, kidney disease, pneumonia/flu, and suicide. Most of these causes are preventable and treatable. Our own lifestyle habits are the largest cause of morbidity; that is, risky behaviors developed in childhood continue throughout adulthood and become various diseases and disorders. Twenty percent of Americans smoke, which causes one out of every five deaths, or 450,000 per year. That's an enormous number.

My previous lifestyle habits were leading me down the path to pre-mature death. I ate refined sugar and "bad" omega-6 fats, did not exercise enough, had high blood pressure, acid reflux, too much visceral fat, almost daily headaches, heart arrhythmias, intestinal cramping, a couple of kidney stones, recurring sharp headaches lasting a brief second, and I was always tired.

Oh, and I had two different cancers.

Boy, did I need a paradigm lifestyle change before I became a statistic! With all this adversity comes opportunity—and ultimately, for me, the very foundation for this book.

In this chapter, we will assemble the Garden of Eden Lifestyle plan to incorporate the four secrets to develop a leaner, stronger body while avoiding cancer and other diseases. The strategy includes the following points:

Create a nutritious diet (not *dieting*) that reduces/eliminates refined sugar and maintains a steady blood insulin level (Secret One).

Utilize the best combination of nutritional supplements to

CHAPTER SIX | THE GARDEN OF EDEN LIFESTYLE

satiate the body and promote the leptin hormone, while inhibiting the ghrelin hormone that induces overeating and hunger pangs (Secret Two).

Employ an intermittent fasting regimen to reduce the total caloric intake; which also increases longevity (Secret Three).

Maintain an exercise program to tone and build muscle while promoting insulin sensitivity of muscle cells so more sugar is absorbed and less is stored as fat (Secret Four).

Before we begin with the process, you will need a baseline starting point. First, take a picture of yourself in a swimsuit so you can see the changes you are about to make. Second, record your clothing sizes and weight. Third, get a blood pressure reading and pulse rate. You may even want to monitor and record the changes in your total body fat.

Total body fat can be determined by using an inexpensive caliper—this method is quite accurate. Some newer digital weight scales can also calculate body fat—they are easier but slightly less accurate. Determination of total body fat provides a number, which represents your percentage of fat present. (See Appendix B for total body fat tables—based on age and gender.) Find the percentage number in the row that matches your age. This will correspond to ranges for lean, ideal, average, and above average people. Note that total body fat values for women are slightly higher, as women naturally carry a little more adipose tissue required for childbearing.

Another method to assess progress utilizes your body mass index (BMI). Note: it has nothing to do with measuring body fat. Body mass index is the value of your mass (weight) divided by the square of your height, or:

$$BMI = weight / height^2$$

Thus, BMI assigns a value to the relationship of your weight and height—used to categorize people into groups.

For a BMI chart that has done the above calculation for you, reference Appendix C. In the chart, line up your weight from the top row, with height in the left column, to find the intersection that gives your BMI number. This chart provides a range for underweight, healthy, overweight, obese, and extremely obese categories—this too can be useful to check progress. Note, however, that BMI does not assess total body fat and the resulting classifications can be misleading. For example, a shorter but bulky muscular person could be considered overweight with BMI values, even though they actually may not have much body fat (as pre-determined by the body fat caliper method). The point is to interpret the data in relative terms.

Your personal recordings give you a starting basis and can help monitor your progress—as well, as provide inspiration. Repeat the measurements monthly to track your improvements.

We will now examine my Garden of Eden Lifestyle's daily and weekly routine, as a working example of how to develop that leaner body you want and deserve. Use this template to create your own Garden of Eden lifestyle. The timing of a routine that works for me may differ for you, depending upon our work schedule and personal preferences; but the important point is to incorporate all the details into a practical and workable plan that resonates with your personal lifestyle.

We will now address diet, supplements, and exercise. Remember to avoid the health hazards discussed in Chapter Five.

CHAPTER SIX | THE GARDEN OF EDEN LIFESTYLE

The Diet

OUR DIET SHOULD be pleasant to eat and easy to prepare, yet effective to provide necessary nutrients for a healthy body. It should include clean water, plus assortment of vegetables and fruits.

In Genesis 1:29, we read:

And God said, Behold, I have given you every herb yielding seed, which is upon the face of all the earth, and every tree, in which is the fruit of a tree yielding seed; to you it shall be for food.

I also highly recommend that you enlist intermittent fasting to limit the total calories consumed, while simultaneously including tasty, but healthy snacks. The best part of the diet is that you choose the food to eat—the ones that *you* like! Fad diets can recommend certain foods, but if you don't like any of them, the fad diet will be just that—a bad fad and a thing of the past, getting you nowhere.

Once you start to follow your healthy, new Garden of Eden Lifestyle diet of eliminating refined sugar, there may be brief episodes of feeling tired and lethargic for a couple of weeks. All due to the transition from a harmful hypoglycemic/hyperglycemic cyclic sugar diet, to one of a low to moderate steady-state sugar-balanced diet. The body is moving from a sugar fuel diet, to a more ketogenic type of diet, complete with healthy omega-3 fats and MCT oil.

After a couple of weeks, the energy you need will return, and you will feel great—that is, as long as you do not "cheat" by eating refined sugars during this time. The best part after this transition is

HEALTHY BODY, HAPPY LIFE

that all fruits and vegetables will taste richer and much better. This is what God provided for humanity—healthy fruits and vegetables that taste great.

Water makes up about 70 percent of the content in the cells of the body. Perspiration, respiration, metabolism, and excretion of water require continual replenishment. Drink only clean water derived from filtering, distillation, or bottling; and be sure that any bottled water is as advertised. When at a local food store, I noticed a man buying five gallons of water from a blue refill machine. From the back of the machine, was a copper water pipe, supplying the refill station. The device "purifies" city water, but to what extent? How often are the filters changed, if at all, to maintain water purity? Who knows? Ask questions!

If you want truly pure water, a distiller is the best answer. It boils water into steam and re-condenses the steam into water, leaving the physical impurities behind. When on vacation, I buy and drink distilled water from the local store—I know the water is truly pure. It does not contain any minerals, but neither does it have harmful impurities. It is also less expensive than the brand-name bottled waters, which may have questionable sources and levels of purity.

Everywhere I go—around the house, in the yard, or in the car—I carry an insulated water bottle with a convenient plastic straw. There is nothing better than ice-cold water, especially on a hot day. The water bottle also goes with me to many social gatherings and serves as a good substitute for other drink options. When thirsty, a few sips or gulps are very satisfying. Often when the brain signals to the body to eat something, what it really needs is water. After taking in water, the hunger sensation disappears. If we were to eat unnecessarily, instead of drinking water, that would

CHAPTER SIX | THE GARDEN OF EDEN LIFESTYLE

add calories and visceral fat, and we would still be thirsty. So drink water first, and if still hungry, then eat something.

Water is always the best choice, but there are many other tempting drinks. Soda pop and fruit juice are poor alternatives; they have a lot of sugar and probably HFCS (high fructose corn syrup). The worst are diet drinks. Artificial sweeteners make you feel hungrier and therefore defeat their intended purpose to reduce calories.

Have you ever wondered what produced the "buzz" from drinking diet soda pop? It is the artificial sweetener acting as an excitotoxin on the brain's glutamate receptors, creating an excitatory state (or buzz); and as we have learned, this chronic stimulation of the brain cells leads to loss of brain function and dementia. The acid in soda pop erodes teeth and inflames the esophagus. A better use for these acidic liquids is cleaning household appliances and surfaces.

At home, our stand-alone icemaker requires periodic cleaning. The manufacturer proposes a chemical that contains both phosphoric and citric acid, but at a high price. Instead, one can use the caramel colored and clear soda pop drinks at a fraction of the cost. Really! They both provide the phosphoric and citric acids, and they do not have to be special ordered and shipped. The local super market will supply them cheaply at most hours of the day.

Keep alcohol consumption to a minimum. There is a reason liquor causes the "beer belly" phenomenon. Alcohol is loaded with calories without many nutritional benefits. It can also lead to unwanted cirrhosis of the liver and cancer. If you already have a debilitating disease or condition, that is another reason to avoid alcohol.

Drink water often and everywhere. A rule of thumb is to drink as much water in ounces as half of your body weight in pounds. Thus, for a 200-pound man, this would be 100 ounces, or about eight, 12-ounce cups of water per day. The 12-ounce cup is the size of a typical kitchen glass. During the summer months, you can even add an electrolyte tablet to the water to help replenish the salts you've lost from sweating. Nuun® makes an "active™" electrolyte tablet that does not have refined sugar and comes in many different flavors.

Eating vegetables and fruits is an integral part of maintaining health. They provide over 5,000 phytonutrients to nourish the body; and remember we can blenderize them to unlock more of their goodness. **Our Garden of Eden Lifestyle Diet** will start with a vegetables/fruits smoothie to begin the daily diet regimen and provide the body with essential nutrients. Since we cannot possibly eat every type of vegetable or fruit, the best ones were elected to yield the most benefit.

All of the produce chosen is organically grown and, when possible, purchased locally. Of course, the best way to ensure the best quality is to grow your own—vine-ripened food always tastes better, too.

The Garden of Eden Lifestyle Smoothie consists of the following vegetables:

    Beets
    Broccoli
    Brussels sprouts
    Red Cabbage
    Carrots

Cauliflower
Celery
Peppers (red, green, or orange)
Tomatoes
Cilantro
Kale
Parsley
Spinach

Peel the beets and wash all the vegetables in a "vegetable wash" to clean off any dirt or residue. I use the Purely Essential Vegetable Wash, obtained online (http://www.purelyessential.com/).

Cut the vegetables into portions about the size of a regular bite of food, except for the cilantro, kale, parsley, and spinach (use the whole bunch). Blanch the cruciferous vegetables: broccoli, Brussels sprouts, cabbage, cauliflower, and kale. Also, blanch the spinach. Freeze the cut vegetables in separate freezer bags for later use.

Blenderize one bunch each of cilantro, kale, parsley, and spinach together in enough water so they puree well. Pour the green mix into plastic ice trays and freeze. Then remove them from the trays and place into plastic freezer bags for frozen storage until needed.

The smoothie also contains the following fruits:

Apples (your choice of variety)
Blueberries
Blackberries
Raspberries
Strawberries

Wash the organic apples and cut into six slices per apple. Freeze them in bags, but try not to let the meat of each slice touch the meat of another as they can be hard to pry apart after frozen; place the skin of the apple next to the meat of another slice. Also freeze the organic blueberries, raspberries, strawberries, and blackberries in separate bags—these are also full of important phyto-nutrients, such as ellagic acid, which have anti-cancer properties. Now we have all the vegetables and fruits prepared and frozen, ready for use. The next step is to combine the ingredients and create our smoothie.

Take seven, 16-ounce glass drinking cups and add one cut frozen portion of each vegetable to each glass. Each portion is about the size of a bite of food. To each glass, add one tablespoon of flaxseed oil, two tablespoons MCT oil, and one-half-teaspoon Concentrace Trace Essential Minerals. Then top it off with one-half- teaspoon of cinnamon. Cinnamon is a powerful antioxidant, and it tastes good. Place plastic wrap over each glass and put them into the refrigerator. *This is your one-week supply.* Note: store the containers of flaxseed and MCT oils in the refrigerator to protect from oxidation.

Every morning, remove one glass of vegetables from the refrigerator and place the contents into the blender container—I personally use the Nutribullet®. Add one frozen green ice-cube of cilantro, kale, parsley, and spinach. Also add ¼ cup frozen blueberries (a great antioxidant); a few each of strawberries, blackberries, and raspberries; and a slice of frozen apple. Add clean water and blenderize.

To create the desired consistency, add water as needed and re-blenderize the mix. I prefer a well-pureed liquid as opposed to a thick mix. This produces two daily requirements of vegetables and

CHAPTER SIX | THE GARDEN OF EDEN LIFESTYLE

fruits in a smoothie mix. *Drink one portion at the start of your daily diet cycle.* With the other portion, you can offer it to your significant other, save it for the evening meal, or save it for the next day. If you have active cancer, it is best to consume the second portion at dinnertime, providing more powerful phytonutrients.

I drink the entire mix all at once, but my wife sips it over time; either way is fine. The taste is not like a gourmet dessert but it is not bad either. The taste buds will adjust to the new flavors, especially after cutting out refined sugar and unhealthy snacks. You may even get to like the taste. Just know, this is the most absolute healthiest drink with over 5,000 phytonutrients, and may just be the closest thing we have to the fountain of youth. Also, realize you are doing your utmost to improve your health and prevent cancer.

So how much does this healthy smoothie cost, $10 . . . $5? The cost of the vegetables and fruits from the local organic market, and the added nutrients from an on-line supplier were inexpensive. The total cost (at the time of this writing) came to $2.85 per day for the *two* servings or just $1.43 per person, for one serving each. Where else can one buy so much organic health for so little?

Lunch occurs any time after the vegetables/fruits smoothie, whenever your schedule allows. It can include various leftovers from dinner, thus it would be considered a brown-bag lunch. However, it does not have to be boring.

My wife makes great dinners, and thus we always have tasty lunches. They often include chicken, low glycemic carbohydrates, and more vegetables.

Everyone's tastes are different so experiment with healthy

choice foods and spices—what satisfies my palate may not be acceptable to yours, and vice versa. Just have fun; and remember to read food labels.

If you work away from home, it is very important not to rely on fast-food restaurants to supply your lunch meals. Do not go to that local burger joint that promises to make your meal happy or give you a whopper of a sandwich deal. Instead, you will just get the double whammy: a dose of heart-killing, artery-congesting deep fried food from omega-6 fats, and a spare tire, "belly-fat", from high glycemic bread and the accompanying HFCS (high fructose corn syrup) soft drink. You will definitely get more than you bargained for in bad health.

Snacks are a great way to tide you over until dinner, but only if they are nutritious. There are many great choices. Organic chips made from non-GMO corn or wheat, with salsa, are tasty treats. Raw nuts, such as macadamia and almonds that provide good omega-3 fats, are good options. If you like coconut, almonds, and chocolate (but only very dark chocolate with high cocoa percentages and without sugar), this triple combination makes a healthy treat very similar to popular candy bars, but without the cancer-inducing sugar. Apples and oranges make good snack food, too.

Just be sure to stay away from tempting foods such as candies, doughnuts, and potato chips. They are loaded with sugar and the bad omega-6 fats.

In addition, remember to drink plenty of water throughout the day as it helps to fill you up and diminish hunger cravings that can lead to unhealthy snack choices.

Dinner is similar to lunch, in that, It's best to eat a good

CHAPTER SIX | THE GARDEN OF EDEN LIFESTYLE

protein source like organic chicken or wild caught salmon, low glycemic complex carbohydrates, and good omega-3 fats. You may have a hamburger or steak now and then, but make sure the animal source is grass-fed and without the injected antibiotics usually found in concentrated animal feeding operations (CAFOs).

It is also best to cut back the use of bread as it contributes to AGE's (advanced glycation end products). This has been hard for me because as a child we always had bread or rolls for dinner. Furthermore, as you know, I enjoyed cake, pie, and ice cream, but I do not eat them regularly now. There are foods that can be healthy substitutes for desserts and help curb the desire for the less beneficial ones. Fortunately, today there are many cookbooks available with healthy recipes to guide your decisions for dinner and dessert alternatives.

Dessert—we all have cravings for a cookie or a small piece of pie with ice cream; and, by all means, you should *occasionally* indulge yourself. Nevertheless, I don't recommend that you make a meal out of dessert, or eat them on a daily basis for weeks on end. The good news is that occasionally eating these foods will not kill you. All the good vegetables, fruits, and supplements counter-balance the adverse effects of these occasional indulgences.

The main point is don't overwhelm your body by continually assaulting it with unhealthy foods. In my opinion, I have found the best substitute for ice cream . . . frozen blue berries! They are cold and have a similar texture to some flavors of ice cream. Best of all, they are antioxidants that are absent of all the refined sugar and fat, so they are extremely healthy.

Experiment with other foods that appeal to your palate: make it fun!

Intermittent fasting is how we bring these basic diet concepts together. Incorporating the Garden of Eden Lifestyle is a critical factor. Out of necessity, our ancient ancestors could only hunt and gather food during daylight hours–and, therefore, they ate only during this limited window of opportunity. Eating during this restricted timeframe kept them from developing excessive visceral fat and obesity due to less total calorie consumption—an unintended but good consequence.

We touched briefly on the timing issues of intermittent fasting. Your work schedule will dictate the pattern that works best for you. The optimal way to determine the best eight-hour window in which to eat depends upon when you go to bed. Stop eating three hours before bedtime. This gives your digestive tract time to digest food and allows for better sleep while not allowing the food to be stored as fat.

From the time you determine when eating stops, calculate eight hours before that, and this becomes the time you will begin to eat during the day. For example, if you plan to go to bed at 10pm that night stop eating by 7pm and begin your eating cycle after 11am of that day.

Do not worry about feeling hungry all the time. When you eat healthy meals, nutritious vegetables and fruits, and take the suggested supplements, you will shift your metabolism into fat-burning mode and have more energy. Besides, the ghrelin hormone will turn off and the leptin hormone will predominate, leaving you satisfied. There have been many days when I forgot to start the eating cycle on time—sometimes it was one or even two hours late. I would then eat only because I knew I needed to, not because my stomach was dying of hunger and growling. What a pleasant change for once!

Another benefit of getting all the necessary daily calories within a circumscribed timeframe is that it eliminates the need to count calories. Frankly, who wants the burden of trying to calculate accurately the calories in various foods—if it is even possible? Eat healthy foods when hungry and drink lots of water; your body will subconsciously tell you to eat more, if needed, or eat less. Our brain signals our body when we need more nutrients; and by eating healthy, wholesome foods, we assure that our body is receiving the proper nutrition.

There are two ways to maintain proper body weight. We can eat just enough nutrients to sustain a healthy weight, or eat in excess, but burn off the excess calories by exercise. We can all agree, it is far easier to maintain the proper body weight by optimal nutrition and supplements than by exercising calories away after the fact. You cannot burn enough calories, especially when you are older, to compensate for an excessive caloric intake that also ages people faster. Besides, eating a lower carbohydrate, good omega-3 fats diet that includes intermittent fasting makes you less hungry.

The diet schedule of my typical Garden of Eden Lifestyle day is basic and consistent. I start with "breakfast" around 11am when I have the vegetables/fruits smoothie. This means I start the day with over 5,000 phyto-nutrients and minerals. An hour or two later, lunch will occur, followed by healthy snacks that I eat whenever the urge arises. Dinner usually happens around 6 pm. That is my eight-hour intermittent fasting diet timeframe. Create your own optimal schedule to benefit your personal needs.

Supplements

SUPPLEMENTS ARE VITAL to overall good health. We will use

the broad term "supplements," but for our purposes, it refers to and includes nutrients, phytonutrients, vitamins, and minerals. The typical American diet doesn't provide sufficient levels of necessary nutrients, especially when we factor in nutrient-depleted soil and contaminated water used to grow our food. If the food supply were more nutritious, we would not see within our population the current levels of obesity or soaring cancer rates. We need to provide the body with essential nutrients to prevent the cravings that lead to overeating—which leads to obesity—and to ward off cancer more effectively. We can avoid the tendency to "super-size" along the way, as we super-energize from the benefit of supplements.

A small confession is in order here. In the introduction, I hinted that you could not take a magic diet pill to lose weight. While that is essentially true, you *can* take supplements to provide the body with the necessary nutrients to satiate the desire to overeat. Therefore, in a sense, this is like taking magic pill<u>s</u>; or, to put it another way, this is God's handiwork–a natural selection of supplements that help create the lean body that God intended for us. Remember, however, that it also takes more than just "popping pills." Diet and exercise are also vital to this reality.

After discovering that the itch above my ear was desmoplastic melanoma, I spent four years studying and researching sites on the internet, scientific studies, journals, and books to find the supplements that best fortify the human body to function at its peak. What I soon realized is that there were significant cross over benefits to healthy diets, supplementation, and exercise. Namely, when the body functions at its optimum, the immune system is enhanced and wards off diseases and especially cancer. However, that was not everything—the best and unexpected aspect found

CHAPTER SIX | THE GARDEN OF EDEN LIFESTYLE

was a leaner, stronger body. This was like winning the lottery while investing just $2.

I often asked myself why nutrition and supplementation weren't taught in school before I had to learn this the hard way. Sadly, in dental school, students earn only 1.4 credit hours for courses on nutrition. Yet, such courses dealt with information directly relating sugar to tooth decay—clearly vital to the work and goals of preventive care dentistry, but not enough. Medical school is not much better. There, physicians receive about 25 credit hours on the subject of nutrition, but only as it relates to other diseases or medications. Naturopaths receive around 60 hours of training in the study of nutrition and supplements, and are thus a better source for answering questions about the necessity of these supplements. Unfortunately, there is still no true Doctoral specialty within the field of medicine to address this growing and indeed desperate need. However, times are changing, and hope remains.

The regimen for taking the supplements, proposed for basic health maintenance and recommended here, is designed for easy remembrance and simple implementation. These nutrients are ingested once daily, even though the dosage information on the bottle may suggest multiple doses taken two to three times daily, or some with food, some without food, some in the morning, some in the evening, or some more often. As you can see, this can get quite confusing and frustrating—which is why I advocate and recommend this more basic approach of once daily. This simplified process means getting the necessary nutrients, though perhaps at a lower dose. Yet this is better than the risk you take at getting none of the necessary supplements because the designated regimen was too hard to follow! Thus, the reasoning is as follows: if the process is easy to perform, you are likely to follow it with consistency; and even lower dosage supplementation is better than none at all. Furthermore, remember you should be getting more of these nutrients naturally from the healthier foods you eat. If you have a special medical condition, disease, or cancer, some vitamins, minerals, and supplements should be increased in dosage and strength to address the ailment. We will examine a few of these examples in Chapter Seven.

Some of you may not be able to take a particular supplement due to potential dangerous interactions with prescription drugs. The goal therefore, would be to get healthier from taking those supplements, which you are able to tolerate, as you wean off the prescription drugs. Ultimately, you want to eliminate prescription drugs, with all their harmful side effects. Nevertheless, I strongly recommend that you first consult with a healthcare practitioner knowledgeable in supplements and drugs before altering your existing program of prescription drug intake.

The following lists of nutrients give the name, dose, type of delivery option, and my preferred brand. The brands of these supplements were determined, in my opinion, to be the best in terms of pill form, bioavailability, other listed ingredients, and cost. Feel free to research and substitute with another brand, as you deem necessary. The detailed information describing the benefits for each supplement has been provided in Chapter Three—please reference that section as needed.

All the information about supplements, vitamins, and minerals and their dosage, applies solely to adult administration. Dosages for children and young adults are not given; please seek the advice of professional healthcare providers for their recommendations.

CHAPTER SIX | THE GARDEN OF EDEN LIFESTYLE

Take these supplements with meals:

Acetyl-L-carnitine 500 mg Vcap, Now®

Aged Garlic Extract 600 mg capsule, Kyolic formula 101®

Alpha Lipoic Acid 250 mg capsule, Now®

Astaxanthin 5 mg softgel, Vitacost®

Biotin 5,000 mcg capsule, Now®

Borage Oil 1300 mg softgel, Vitacost®

Calcium with magnesium and vitamin D3, Rainbow Light®

Ginkgo Biloba 120 mg Vcap, Now®

Grape Seed Extract 100 mg Vcap, Now®

Green Tea Extract (EGCg) 400 mg capsule, Now®

Hawthorn extracts 1000 mg per serving, capsule, Vitacost®

L-Carnosine 500 mg capsule, Vitacost®

Magnesium malate 1250 mg (three tablets yield 425 mg magnesium), Source Naturals®

Max DHA 560 mg per serving, softgel, Jarrow®

5MTHF (methyl folate) 1 mg capsule, Thorne®

NAC (N-acetyl cysteine) 600 mg capsule, Now®

Niacinamide 500 mg capsule, Nature's Way®

Probiotic 10-20 (20 billion) capsule, Vitacost®

Pycnogenol (pine bark extract) 50 mg capsule, Vitacost®

Quercetin and Bromelain 500 mg capsule, Vitacost®

Toco-Sorb (tocotrienols) softgel, Jarrow®

Trans Resveratrol 500 mg capsule, Vitacost®

Turmeric Force (curcumin) 400 mg softgel, New Chapter ®

Ubiquinol 100 mg softgel, Now®

Unique E—400 IU softgel, Grace ®

Vitamin B 12-methylcobalamine 5,000 mcg capsule, Vitacost®

Vitamin D3 5,000 IU softgel, Vitacost®

Vitamin K w/ K2 complex, Vitacost®

Vinpocetine 10 mg, capsule, Vitacost®

Take these supplements before breakfast (or between meals):

Carotenall (mixed carotenoids) softgel, Jarrow®

CLA (conjugated linoleic acid) 800 mg softgel, Now®

L-Arginine 500 mg capsule, Now®

PQQ 10 mg capsule, Vitacost®

Taurine 500 mg capsule, Now®

Active senior multivitamin tablet, Rainbow Light®, (men's one or women's one)

Liposomal C --1000 mg (vitamin C) capsule, two times daily, Dr. Mercola Premium Supplements®

Take this supplement before bed:

Melatonin 5 mg Vcap, Now®

CHAPTER SIX | THE GARDEN OF EDEN LIFESTYLE

Take this supplement before breakfast, once per week as a maintenance dose (or daily for 2-3 weeks while fighting active infections such as a cold or flu):

Beta 1,3/1,6 Glucan capsule, Now®

You may think this is a huge list of supplements; and yes, it is! My mother, who is 85, jokingly says she is starting to look like a supplement capsule walking down the street (I picture a cartoon character looking like a pill with two arms and legs strolling along the sidewalk). However, she doesn't look like a capsule just yet. She will also tell you that she feels so much better and has more energy while taking the supplements and drinking her daily smoothie. In addition, she has lost weight!

It is necessary to take these supplements because our Western American diet does not provide all the nutrients we need. Even with the volume of supplements listed, it is less expensive than prescription drugs that would otherwise be required had we gotten sick. It's healthier, too. The cost of medical care and time off from work are other factors we must consider.

A report claims people aged 45 and older take an average of four prescription drugs. The average cost of one brand-name drug in 2013, was nearly 3000 dollars ($2,960, to be precise) per year. This totals almost 12,000 dollars ($11,840) per year per person for just four prescription drugs. The average cost for healthcare in 2012 was almost 9,000 dollars ($8,915), while the cost of time lost from taking leave for being sick in 2003, for all Americans, totaled 260 billion dollars.

By adding these numbers together, it is clear that the cost of being ill is enormous. It is much less expensive and more prudent to maintain a healthy lifestyle to prevent disease in the first place.

The increased energy, better mental acuity, and comfort of knowing that your body is able to function at peak performance while preventing atherosclerosis, cardiovascular disease, diabetes, dementia, and especially cancer is well worth the relatively modest price of the supplements. So now, you ask, just how much do all these supplements cost? To take all of them—about 40 supplements—costs about $5.88 per day at the time of this writing, or about $0.16 per supplement. That is just over 2,000 dollars per year ($2,146). This is five times less than the cost of the prescription drugs alone, which does not even include the savings for healthcare costs and time lost from work. Wouldn't you agree that $5.88 per day is well worth the price for physical, emotional, and psychological well-being?

Thank God that Big Pharma cannot patent these nutrients—because, believe me they would if they could; and the price would then skyrocket. Since they are natural or plant-based in origin, this prohibits Big Pharma from monopolizing supplements via a patent, which would then allow them to extract enormous profits at the expense of the consumers.

What about the safety issues with prescription drugs? The DEA (Drug Enforcement Agency) announced on November 4, 2015, in their National Drug Threat Assessment (NDTA) report, that death by drug overdose is the leading cause of injury death in the U.S., which is more than deaths from motor vehicle accidents and firearms. These facts rely on 2013 statistics where more than 46 thousand people died in the U.S. from drug overdoses. More than half of the drug overdoses were due to prescription painkillers and heroin. We need an alternative to dangerous prescription drugs; luckily, we have non-prescription supplements.

CHAPTER SIX | THE GARDEN OF EDEN LIFESTYLE

Here are a few suggestions for purchasing and organizing the supplements. There are many online supplement companies, but I buy my supplements from Vitacost®.com and have them shipped to my doorstep. This saves a lot of time and money. Vitacost® frequently offers many supplements on sale, which reduces the cost stated above. For even further cost reduction, buy the largest quantities for the better price break—the volume discount approach.

To make sure to get the best value on the purchase of supplements, I maintain a supplement inventory system that alerts me when to replenish the dwindling supplements and take advantage of sale prices. I retain a four-drawer system in the kitchen to store the supplement bottles. There is a drawer for those taken before breakfast/between meals, and its backup drawer. In addition, there is another drawer for those taken with meals, and their backup drawer. The two primary drawers have one bottle of each supplement to make up each week's daily allotment, while the backup drawers are to maintain inventory and resupply the primary drawer when a particular supplement runs out. This way I purchase the supplements on sale and store them until needed, and there is never a worry of running out of stock.

To make up the week's supply of supplements have separate drawers for each person taking them. I have a drawer for my wife and one for myself—this is important because the needs of the person can vary and men and women will not take the same multi-vitamin, since they are gender specific. .

Place 14 paper-drinking cups in each person's drawer, seven cups for supplements taken "before breakfast/between meals", and seven cups for those taken "with meals". Dispense one "before breakfast/between meals" supplement into each of the seven cups for use during the week. After all are dispersed, take a sandwich baggy and place the cup contents of supplements into the bag, remove as much air as possible, and seal it, and put the baggy back into the cup; this helps maintain freshness and minimizes their oxidation. Repeat the process for the "with meals supplements". It is now easier in the morning to grab a baggy from the "before breakfast/between meals" cup and a baggy from the "with meals" cup, and take the supplements to work. Then take them at the appropriate time during the day.

The Beta Glucan capsule is placed in only one cup of the "before breakfast/between meals" for maintenance dosing. If you have an active infection, place one Beta Glucan in every cup for two weeks to stimulate the immune system. For the melatonin, place the bottle in your bathroom or nightstand, so you can take it 30 minutes before bed.

Here is a note about probiotics and supplements that contain any oil, like Borage, curcumin, DHA, CLA, and softgels; refrigerate these to prolong the shelf life. If refrigeration is not possible, just keep them in a cool area out of direct sunlight. While on vacation, take supplements with you and refrigerate them; but do not panic if that is not possible, the oxidation to the oils will be minimal if kept cool and out of direct sunlight.

As previously discussed, the toxic levels for supplements are much higher than the dosages suggested on the bottle. However, this does not mean you cannot develop intolerance to one, the most common of which is diarrhea, but again usually at extreme doses. The supplements that can cause diarrhea at high doses are vitamin C, vitamin D3, vitamin E, curcumin, DHA, gingko biloba, hesperidin, magnesium, niacinamide, probiotics, pycnogenol, and taurine.

If by chance intolerance is experienced, stop taking the supplements until the diarrhea subsides and then reintroduce them one at a time. If the diarrhea re-appears, the culprit will show itself. This happened to me with Hesperidin. After long-term use, my body grew intolerant to Hesperidin and I discovered it by the re-introduction process. I have not had a problem since, or with any others.

The supplement schedule is based off the intermittent fasting schedule. Since my eating schedule is from 11am to 7pm, I take my "before breakfast/between meals" supplements after I get up in the morning, well before 11am. A glass of water is also beneficial to flush out the kidneys and toxins that accumulated overnight.

I take the "with meals" supplements usually after the vegetables/fruits smoothie is consumed around 11am, or after lunch. This gets more nutrients into the body and staves off any hunger throughout the day. Finally, the melatonin is taken 30 minutes before bed.

How should one consume the numerous supplements? The "before breakfast/between meals" nutrients are few and I take them together. If you cannot do that, separate them into smaller quantities. The "with meals" supplements can be daunting. Ingest the "sinkers" together and after separating them from the "floaters". Then take the "floaters" in either two or three separate portions, depending upon your preferences. With practice, you'll get them down.

Exercise

EXERCISE IS EXTREMELY beneficial to tone and build muscle,

along with so many more benefits to the body. It produces human growth hormone (HGH), and strengthens the heart. Exercise also burns excess calories by exhausting blood glucose stores, while reducing the risk of diabetes.

Exercise can take on many forms, from walking, jogging, running, swimming, dancing, sporting activities, weight training, Pilates, treadmills, aerobics, and anything that gets you moving. The best routine will incorporate moderate weights using high-intensity strength training (HIST) and high-intensity interval training (HIIT). Another wonderful result is that toned muscles will keep joints healthy and in alignment, reducing the need for chiropractic manipulation or physical therapy.

The full body workout routine that follows is the one I use to take advantage of HIIT and HIST, without resulting in extreme fatigue or exhaustion. You should feel good after the workout, the result of the released endorphins' effect on the brain. In addition, one may notice having a warmer, body-core temperature than usual. This may last for hours after the routine due to increased cellular metabolism and the burning of fat stores while building muscle fibers.

Note that most of these exercise routines appear on YouTube, where proper form is illustrated. If you have any physical limitations, seek advice from a personal trainer. You may want, or need, to alter your routine to obtain the ultimate results you desire. Just follow the basic principles and adapt the regimen to meet those needs. My personal goal for the regimen is for total body muscle tone with some bulk added. The routine is the accumulation of many different exercise programs, followed over the years, with the best aspect of each retained and incorporated herein.

The HIST Routine

THIS INVOLVES THE use of free weights. In the beginning, use lighter weights or even none at all. Then gradually increase the weight after you have mastered the form and can execute each exercise properly.

One can perform this exercise program in a fitness center or at home. If done at home, you'll need to obtain a few items to facilitate your workout. You will need a set of free weights (dumbbells), a mat (or thick rug), an inflatable exercise ball, and a battery operated clock with a second hand (or cell phone with a clock; but do not place it close to your body).

Starting out, you may want to complete only two sets of any exercise for the first week or two. That's fine. Add the third set when you feel able, and eventually add the fourth and final set. Only after you are comfortable with doing four sets should you gradually increase the weights. It is much better to perform these exercises correctly, with lighter weights, than to injure yourself. Give yourself all the time you need—we are not in a hurry! Listen to your body to guide you: if your muscles are sore, give yourself longer recovery intervals. In time, you will develop your routine at four sets per exercise at your appropriate weight. I would rather see you develop the regimen smartly and effectively than to become frustrated and burn out from having overdone things—only to stop entirely. I want you to succeed—I am with you in spirit all the way!

1) **Warm-up**—it is important to get the heart pumping faster and the core body warmed up a few degrees. A slow to moderate pace on the elliptical machine, jumping jacks, or running in place will increase your core temperature and get the blood flowing

better. This helps prevent injury to muscles and joints. Then stretch to loosen muscles. Note: it is best to stretch before running, doing sprints, or performing HIIT. However, stretching before HIST can be counterproductive and decrease your strength performance; just make sure you warm-up first.

The best exercise to start the HIST routine is one that works on the quadriceps (quads) or thigh muscles. This is the largest muscle group. Reports show that doing arm curls after squats results in more bulk obtained in the biceps because the quad workout stimulates more blood flow and releases human growth hormone to the entire body.

2) **Squats**—place the feet slightly wider apart than shoulder width, with toes pointed slightly outward. Keep your back in a neutral position, as vertical as possible, with the stomach tucked in. The balance through the motion should be more on the heel of the feet; this also keeps the knees centered over the feet. Knees too far forward cause injury to the knee joint.

Use a dumbbell of appropriate weight in each hand, with the arms straight down and over the thighs. Slowly bend the knees until the upper and lower leg form a 90-degree angle, all while moving the dumbbell weights forward just in front of the knees. This acts as a counter balance and maintains better form with the knees not extending past the toes. Now return to the starting position. That comprises one repetition.

Slowly bend the knees for a count of three, while inhaling through the nose. Then stand up or extend the legs for a count of one while exhaling through the nose. It takes four seconds to do one repetition; and since we do 10 reps (reps is the short term for repetitions), this will take 40 seconds to complete. The four-second count is as follows: Bending the knees will be for counts 1, 2, 3

CHAPTER SIX | THE GARDEN OF EDEN LIFESTYLE

and then standing will be the completion of the first rep, so then count 1 to designate one completed rep. For the second rep, the count would be 1,2,3,2; followed by 1,2,3,3; and 1,2,3,4; then 1,2,3,5; 1,2,3,6 ……1,2,3,9; and lastly 1,2,3,10. This is one way to count the repetitions per set. If another method to count reps works better for you, by all means, use it.

We will do four sets of 10 reps each and rest 40 seconds between sets. On the last set, do as many as possible with proper form. Note that improper form due to fatigue can lead to injury—always maintain proper form. When starting out learning and performing the exercises, rest 40 seconds between sets by using the clock for timing. However, as you feel more comfortable and after building endurance, there is another option.

Instead of standing around for 40 seconds between sets, we can use that time to perform another exercise for 40 seconds and effectively alternate between the two exercises. This truly makes this a HIST workout. In this case we will use a different muscle group entirely—the arms and shoulders, so we do not conflict with the work on the quads.

3) **Push-ups**—with the hands at shoulder width, lower your body until the chest is close to the floor, or the elbows are at a 90-degree angle. Lower for a count of three while inhaling, and push up for one second while exhaling. Do 10 reps per set and four sets—the count management system is similar to squats. Push-ups strengthen the triceps muscle and upper torso.

In the beginning, you may want to modify the push-up to make it easier, until you generate more strength. One possibility, start by performing the traditional push-up while on the knees instead of feet. Another option is to do the push-ups against the wall, with your feet away from the wall as far as possible. Then, as your strength increases, do the push-ups with your hands on a stable desk, then maybe a chair, and move eventually to the floor. To transition from the chair to the floor, I built a layered platform—using some 2X6 wood scraps—to perform the push-ups. As my strength increased, I removed one board at a time.

Since 10 push-ups take 40 seconds, we can do them between the quad sets. Therefore, the sequence is quads, push-ups, quads, push-ups, quads, push-ups, quads, push-ups—done with both muscle groups. Again, starting out, you may elect to rest during the 40-second rest periods. Now, it is on to the biceps curl.

4) **Biceps curl**—I use dumbbells to take excessive pressure off the wrists and elbows. Start with the dumbbells at your side and parallel to each other. Raise your arms to the chest while rotating the hands 90-degrees. Then lower the arms while rotating the hands to the original starting position. That completes one rep.

Perform four sets of ten reps, with the fourth set done to muscle fatigue; in other words, do as many as possible with proper form on the last set.

When executing the curl, breathe out while raising the bar for a count of one, and breathe in while lowering it for a count of three—and remember to always breath through the nose to increase the nitric oxide levels. Here the count management is still 1,2,3,1; 1,2,3,2; 1,2,3,3; 1,2,3,4 and so forth, until you reach 1,2,3,9; 1,2,3,10. The only difference here is that the short one-second count is on 1 and not the last number, which signifies the total reps.

With a little practice, the different routines with their unique counts will become second nature; just be patient.

Also important, fully lower the dumbbells so the arms are

straight; this creates a full contraction of the muscle through its full range of motion. In this way, more muscle fibers contract, producing more bulk more quickly. This also allows you to employ lighter weights, which puts less strain on the joints.

When doing curls, weight train for 40 seconds, then rest between sets for 40 seconds by monitoring the clock.

Another option, as before, is to perform a different exercise during the rest phase of the biceps curl process that doesn't use the same muscles. In this case, the military press works well.

5) **Military press**—with the dumbbells starting at shoulder level and palms straight out, press them up over your head and bring them slightly together without touching. This is for the count of one while breathing out. Then lower the weights back to shoulder level for a count of three while breathing in. That is one rep; do ten reps per set and four sets. Again, do as many reps on the last set as possible while maintaining proper form. The count management is the same as for the biceps curl.

6) **Bent-over rows**—use dumbbells with the palms facing the body. Slightly bend the knees, and maintain a straight back (no arching) while bending at the waist so that the back almost parallel with the floor. The arms will hang straight down, with back muscles fully extended and relaxed. While not moving the torso, lift the arms (with the elbows perpendicular to the body) up as far as possible while pulling the shoulder blades together. The action is similar to rowing a boat and hence the name. Breathe out for a count of one. Now slowly lower the dumbbells for a count of three while exhaling, until the arms fully extend downward. This is one rep.

Do four sets of ten reps, with the fourth set performed to

muscle fatigue while maintaining proper form. With this exercise, you may do upright row sets during the rest phase of the bent-over rows, or elect to rest the 40 seconds. Do whichever option you are most comfortable; however, combining exercises shortens the overall length of the time to perform all exercises.

7) **Upright rows**—using dumbbells in each hand, start with the arms in front, palms facing the body, with the back straight. Raise the dumbbells close to the body as you exhale for a count of one. At the peak, the dumbbells should almost touch your chin while the elbows will be higher than the forearms. Now lower them back to the thighs, while inhaling, for a count of three. This is one repetition; do 10 reps per set. Perform four sets in between the bent-over row sets, or with a separate rest phase. As always, perform the fourth set to muscle fatigue while maintaining proper form.

Do not jerk or swing the dumbbells as this could cause rotator cuff injury—always use the proper weight and form.

This concludes the standing portion of the workout. Now we will focus more on the core muscle groups. The core routine presented includes my personal preferences, but you can modify it to your needs. Many of the exercises involve static or motionless tension (isometric), to tone and strengthen the slow-twitch fibers of the core. Grab your mat, or thick rug, and the clock. Set the clock on the floor so the second hand is visible for timing some of these exercises.

8) **The plank**—is just as it sounds; you make a rigid plank out of your body and hold it. On the mat, get on your elbows and toes with the legs and back making a straight line parallel to the floor. Hold this position for 90 seconds. For those starting out, begin with a reduced time, say 15 seconds, and add time as the muscle

strength increases. Alternatively, start out by making a plank from knees to elbows and progress from there.

When finished stay on the mat. Get on your hands and knees, and keep the back parallel to the floor.

9) **Cross leg/arm** extensions—this is a yoga move to strengthen the core and improve balance. Start with the right arm and left leg by slowly extending both straight out and then up as far as possible, both at the same time. The movement of both limbs must be coordinated to maintain balance. Keep the arm straight at the elbow and raise it slowly as high as possible. Feel the contraction of the deltoid muscle in the shoulder. At the same time, extend the leg backwards while pointing the toes. Raise the straight leg as high as possible; this strengthens and tones the gluteus maximus muscle for a better-looking backside.

Perform one set of eight repetitions for each limb for a total count of 16. Then reposition on the mat for another core strengthening exercise.

10) **The side plank**—is similar to the regular plank, but done on your side. Execute both right and left sides for 30 seconds each. Start by lying on either side, with the elbow directly under the shoulder. Now straighten and raise the mid-section to form the side plank. You are essentially contacting the ground with the elbow and feet. The opposite arm is at either the side or straight up in the air for balance. After 30 seconds, switch sides to tone the opposite area.

A variation of the side plank involves free arm and hand. Place the hand under the chest near the elbow contacting the floor. The arm is essentially across the torso. Then raise the arm straight up. As you raise and lower the arm, follow the arm with your head

HEALTHY BODY, HAPPY LIFE

so you can always see your hand. This develops more core muscles in a dynamic fashion. Do as many reps as possible in 30 seconds. Switch sides and repeat the process.

Now grab an exercise ball. The inflatable exercise ball comes in three basic sizes: small (purple), medium (blue), and large (green). Technically, the size coincides toward a small, medium, or large person; but my wife (at 5'4") and I (at 6'1") both use the medium size blue exercise ball. Again, use what is most comfortable.

Place your buttocks on the edge of the mat with the feet extending away from the mat. Lie on your back and extend the arms away from the body touching the floor to create stability during the next couple of exercises.

11) **Reverse plank leg curl with ball**—with the exercise ball off the mat, rest both feet on top of it about shoulder length apart. Raise your mid-section to form a straight line from the feet to the shoulders resting on the mat. This forms the reverse plank.

During the exercise, pull the toes toward the knees to contract and tone the shin muscles. Now with the heels of the feet, pull the ball toward you by contracting the hamstring muscles, to where the knees form a 90-degree angle. Contract the hamstrings for a count of one, and then extend the legs so the ball rotates away from the body, for a count of three. Do 16 reps, and then while still in the full reverse plank position, remain in a stationary position for a count of 24.

12) **Wide leg scissors with ball**—with the arms still to the side for balance, drop each foot to the side of the ball, in the middle. With straight legs, pick the ball up off the floor with the feet and rotate the ball by doing leg scissors, or raising one leg

while lowering the other. Do this to a count of 24, or 12 reps per leg.

13) **Ball sit-ups or crunches**—on top of the exercise ball while on your back, arch fully backwards to stretch the abdominal muscles (abs) before performing the crunch. Rise as high as possible to contract the abs for a count of one second, then slowly lower the shoulders and arch backwards to the starting position during a count of three seconds. Breathe out while contracting, and in while extending; do 16 repetitions.

We are now done with the exercise ball, so put it away.

The next exercise is a combination of moves to target the pectoralis major and minor muscles (chest muscles) and the abdominal muscles. Grab two sets of dumbbells—one medium, and one heavier weight. Lie on the mat face up with the knees bent at 90 degrees. Grab the lighter dumbbells first.

14) **Chest fly with abdominal crunch**—raise the dumbbells up over the body with the arms at a 45-degree angle with the floor and directed toward the feet. Keep the elbows slightly bent. Lower the dumbbells straight out from the side, just above the floor for a count of one second, and raise them again to the starting position again for another count of one second. While raising the dumbbells back to the starting position, perform an abdominal crunch. The 45-degree angle of the arms engages more upper chest and shoulder muscles—pectoralis and deltoids.

That is one rep. Do 24 reps while breathing in upon lowering and breathing out upon raising the dumbbells and abdominal crunch. After the last rep, lower the arms straight out to the side just off the floor (while keeping the elbows slightly bent) and hold for 16 seconds.

Now grab the heavier dumbbells.

15) **Chest press**—the dumbbells start in line straight over the chest about shoulder width apart. Lower them until the elbows make a 90-degree angle, for a count of one second. Now press the weights back above the body to the starting position; this also takes one second. Do 24 reps while breathing out during contraction of the muscles, or pushing the weights up and away from the body. Breathe in while lowering the weights. This engages the main middle chest muscles—pectoralis major and minor. You may have wondered why we do 24 repetitions. This number of reps still works on the fast-twitch muscles, but the lighter weight exerts less harmful stress on the shoulder joint and rotator cuff.

Now raise the dumbbells over head for the starting position for the next exercise.

16) **Floor triceps curl**—raise both arms and weights straight up and over the body. The weights are now parallel. With the upper arm rigid, bend one arm at the elbow and bring the dumbbell close to the ear until the elbow is at 90 degrees. Just do not hit your ear, it does not feel good—I know, I tried it . . . Twice. Then raise the dumbbell back to the starting position. Alternate now and do the other arm. Do 12 reps with each arm or 24 total. Now grab the lighter dumbbells for the second half of the chest exercises.

17) **Chest fly with leg lift**—this is the same chest fly as before, except the angle of the arms start over the body 45 degrees toward and over the head. Keep the elbows slightly bent. Lower the dumbbells straight out to the side of the body, just above the floor with a count of one second, and raise them again to the starting position with another count of one second. Another difference is that we will not do a crunch, but will do straight leg lifts while raising the dumbbells. Starting out you may want to

CHAPTER SIX | THE GARDEN OF EDEN LIFESTYLE

raise one leg at a time and as an alternative raise both legs at the same time. Make sure to keep the knees slightly bent.

The 45-degree angle of the arms engages the lower pectoralis and even the latissimus dorsi (side) muscle. Do 24 reps while breathing in upon lowering and breathing out upon raising the dumbbells with the leg lift. After the last rep, lower the arms to the side just off the floor and hold for 16 seconds.

Now grab the heavier dumbbells.

18) **Chest press**—done the same as before with 24 reps.

19) **Floor triceps curl**—also done as before with 24 reps.

Set the weights down. It is time for a little stretching to prevent rotator cuff injuries. While on the mat face up, raise the right arm straight into the air. Let it drift to the left toward the left shoulder. With the left hand, grab behind the right elbow and gently pull the right arm to the left shoulder. You should notice a stretch in the outer area of the right shoulder. Do not bounce or use excessive force. Switch arms and repeat the steps. Stay there on the mat for more abdominal exercises.

20) **Crunches**—these are the typical crunches with the shoulders lifted up off the floor for a count of one second, and then lowered back to the floor for a count of one second. Place the hands behind the head for support, but do not pull on the neck or head. Make sure to contract abdominal muscles while raising the shoulders. Do 16 reps with the shoulders returning to the floor each time.

Next, with the shoulders continually off the floor as high as you can, do 16 mini crunches with the up and down movement for a count of one second. Follow this up with the shoulders continually off the floor and the abs contracted continually for a count of 16. All three of these crunch exercises engage the three different types of core muscle fibers: slow-twitch type I fibers, fast-twitch type IIa fibers and fast-twitch type IIb fibers. Knowing muscle fiber physiology helps to incorporate correct exercises for each fiber type.

Remain in the same position. We will perform a crossover variation of the crunch.

21) **Crossover crunches**—start in the basic crunch position; shoulders on the floor with the hands resting behind the head, elbows to the side, and the legs bent at the knees. Begin the crossover crunch by taking the right shoulder and elbow across the body toward the left leg, while simultaneously lifting the left bent leg up toward the right shoulder. After the crunch, the right shoulder returns to the starting position while straightening the left leg down and away from the body, while keeping it six inches off the floor. That is one rep; do 16 total reps for the right shoulder. Then repeat with 16 reps for the left shoulder and right leg. For good measure, go back to the right shoulder/left leg and then the left shoulder/right leg. You have now completed 64 crossover crunches.

Reposition on your left side while still on the mat. The next exercise works more on the abdominal side muscles.

22) **Side crunch raises**—these are the same as abdominal crunches except that the starting and ending points are while lying on your side. Start with either side. With the hands behind the head for support, raise the upper torso off the mat as far as possible, for a count of one. Now lower to the floor for a one count. Do a total of 16 reps. You should feel the opposite side oblique and transverse muscles contract during this exercise.

As with the regular crunches, we will do 16 mini side crunches. Follow that with a continual side crunch for a count of 16. Then turn over and repeat the steps for the other side. Now lie on your back for more regular abdominal crunches.

23) **Crunches**—repeat the typical crunch regimen (see 20. above). Then, while still lying on your back we will do the last crunch exercise.

24) **Rope pull crunch**—keep the legs bent with the feet on the floor. Pretend you have a rope hanging from the sky with the end touching your belly button. Reach as high as you can with the right hand to grab the imaginary rope and pull yourself up by contracting the abdominal muscles. Then alternate by reaching up as high as possible with the left hand to pull yourself up. Go back and forth until you have done 12 reps per side, or 24 altogether. Go ahead and reach for the stars. We are almost done with the core.

25) **The plank**—we started with the plank and we will end with it too. This time do the plank for 60 seconds. Your core should feel like it has had a good workout, as well as the rest of the body.

Wow, that felt great; and the good news is that it took less than 60 minutes to complete. The best news is yet to come. It is now time for some protein. However, this is just not any protein drink. How does an ice-cold, thick protein shake sound?

The protein shake—this nutritional drink is recommended after the exercise regimen. It is crucial to consume protein within an hour after exercising, giving the muscles the proper building blocks to form new fibers. This shake consists of ice, water, Orgain Organic Protein™ (comes in vanilla or chocolate), MCT oil, blueberries, blackberries, strawberries, and raspberries, a Nuun®

HEALTHY BODY, HAPPY LIFE

electrolyte tablet, plus an optional touch of Cinnamon for a little spice.

Place crushed ice in the Nutribullet® plastic mixing container so it is one-third full. Add water to cover the ice by one-half inch. Pour in two tablespoons of MCT oil. Then add a small golf-ball size of each berry (except for blueberries where I add a half cup due to their antioxidant protection), the electrolyte tablet, cinnamon, and cover the contents with one heaping scoop of the protein powder. Screw the mixing blades into the plastic jar and shake to mix all the contents together. Now place plastic container on the Nutribullet® to blenderize the contents and chop the ice to create a uniform consistency. This usually takes about 30 seconds. Now you have a thick creamy shake to enjoy while you provide your body with protein to build stronger muscles.

Each component of this protein has a specific purpose. The ice makes the drink cold like a thick milkshake. The MCT oil provides medium chain fatty acids to supply ketone bodies for brain fuel while making the shake thick and creamy. The berries provide antioxidants and ellagic acid, known cancer inhibitors. The Nuun® tablet helps replace lost electrolytes and the fizz makes the shake taste interesting. In addition, the cinnamon has antioxidant properties, and adds flavor.

Note that this product has no GMO's, no added sugar, no MSG, is low in natural sugar content, is organic, and has dietary fiber. Now let us look at the protein content. This plant-based protein provides a wide array of amino acids. Here is a list of the amino acids and the amount supplied in one serving:

Alanine	1210 mg
Arginine	1690 mg

Asparagine/Aspartic Acid	1860 mg
Cysteine/Cystine	388 mg
Glutamine	3610 mg
Glycine	902 mg
Histidine	449 mg
Isoleucine	997 mg
Leucine	1770 mg
Lysine	829 mg
Methionine	534 mg
Phenylalanine	1190 mg
Proline	975 mg
Serine	1040 mg
Threonine	759 mg
Tryptophan	185 mg
Tyrosine	1220 mg
Valine	1220 mg

The three amino acids most important for building muscle are the branched chain amino acids isoleucine, leucine, and valine. These three combine for around four grams, or about 20 percent of the total content. It can't get any better than this—tasty, healthy, thick and creamy, and muscle-enhancing. This shake makes me want to work out right now!

The HIIT Routine

HIIT IS THE counterpart to HIST. It is the aerobic exercise element that makes this exercise regimen complete. The principle is simple: exert intense physical output for 30 seconds, followed by light output for 90 seconds. Perform eight cycles, and that is it—done. This takes about 20 minutes from warm-up to cool down.

We have already seen the science behind the benefits of HIIT over traditional cardio workouts in Chapter Four. Let's decide when "to do a HIIT" (no pun intended—but don't say this to a police officer).

I prefer to do a HIIT between strength training (HIST) days. This does a couple of things. First, it makes all workouts shorter because the workouts occur over more days. Second, it allows you to exert more effort per workout, as there is less total fatigue than if HIIT and HIST occurred on the same day. This also maintains a higher level of metabolism for longer periods—thus, it is better for controlling hyperglycemia and diabetes while promoting weight loss.

The elliptical trainer makes a great machine for HIIT, especially if it also has the arm attachments. It can be programmed to create various ramp angles and resistance thereby giving everyone an individualized and unique workout.

As mentioned before, HIIT can be done while running in place and moving your arms (maybe with very light dumbbells) for 30 seconds. If a swimming pool is available, swim hard with your favorite swim stroke. If you are close to a track, running fast for 30 seconds while walking for 90 seconds also works. Whatever you do, make it fun.

Your Exercise Schedule

THIS DEPENDS ON personal needs and desires. Some people may want to work out in the morning, others midday, and yet others in the evening. Schedule a time of day that works best for you, and make it a habit. The days of the week to work out are also variable. Both HIST and HIIT should be done two to three times weekly depending on the results you desire. If you want toned muscles, do them twice weekly, but if you want more bulk do them three times weekly. You can do them on the same day or different days. The advantage of alternating between the two on different days is to provide the body a recovery period, while keeping the exercise time under an hour. My preference is as follows: HIST on Monday, Wednesday, and Friday, and HIIT on Tuesday, Thursday, and again Saturday, with Sunday off.

Alternatively, I may take Wednesday as another recovery day and do HIST on Thursday and HIIT on Friday. The third set of HIST and HIIT totally depends on my home schedule (and maybe even the honey-do-list), so I might not get to it at all. However, that's okay. I'm getting the results I need and want. My goals are for full body muscle tone with slight bulking up of a few muscle groups. Your needs will likely be different, so do what is best to accomplish your own personal goals for getting in shape.

Another reason I may not implement the third set of HIST/HIIT is that I get plenty of exercise from other activities. My wife and I walk during most lunch hours (except when it rains) and this provides additional exercise. We take care of errands during the walks, or just get a change of scenery from working inside a building all day. Try to walk as much as possible—it will even save on gasoline expenses. We are also active in growing and cultivating our organic garden. This provides all our fresh vegetables and fruits for the smoothies, clean air to breathe, and physical exercise—all that the body needs!

There is some disagreement about how many weeks to work out before taking a week off to let the body recover and rest. Some fitness experts say to tone down the routine for a week every so often, and others say to take a half week off every now and then. Clearly, this isn't exactly a scientific designation! In this regard, listen to your body and do what seems right for you. Personally, I shoot for eight to twelve weeks, then take off a whole week, arranging the week off around vacations or holidays when possible. When returning to the exercise program, I recommend that you take it easy the first week back by using lighter weights—do not rush and cause unnecessary joint injury or muscle pain.

There is also disagreement about whether to eat or not before a workout. In essence, it depends upon the intensity of the exercise routine that day and how you feel. For the shorter time needed to complete a HIIT session, eating beforehand is not critical. Just know you will deplete the blood stream of available quick glucose energy. This should not be a problem, since that is one goal of cardio exercise—to lose weight and visceral fat by burning carbohydrates.

The problem occurs when performing intense HIST routines to improve muscle bulk or speed. In this case, a light snack of coconut oil, MCT oil, or raw nuts for energy will achieve that result. Just do not go overboard with sugary snacks. Eat these energy fats 30 minutes before the workout so they are available for metabolism by the muscle cells. The protein shake afterward provides the nutrients to build bulk muscle–and remember to drink a lot of water to aid in cellular metabolism.

CHAPTER SIX | THE GARDEN OF EDEN LIFESTYLE

The Total Time Commitment to Implement The Garden Of Eden Lifestyle Plan

PREPARING HEALTHY VEGETABLES/FRUITS and protein smoothies, managing the supplements, and exercising, is not as time consuming as one might think. To prepare the smoothies takes about eight hours per month. Ordering and organizing the supplements takes about four hours per month. Exercising takes about 16 hours per month. Altogether, it takes about 28 hours per month, or less than one hour per day, and costs less than $10 per person per day to live a healthy Garden of Eden Lifestyle. That is well worth the price to have a healthy body, happy life.

Another way to look at this is to ask yourself, "how much time do I spend watching TV every day?" The average person watches about five hours every day. What if we took one of those TV hours and committed it to our health instead? Better yet, consider preparing the smoothies, organizing the supplements, and exercising *while watching TV*. That's a bonus where we still watch TV but get healthier doing it!

Conclusion

PHIL'S DESMOPLASTIC MELANOMA involved the "perfect storm" for developing cancer. He drank a lot of soda pop with high fructose corn syrup. He absorbed large amounts of MSG and nitrates from eating processed meats, potato chips, and French fries from fast-food restaurants. Phil also over-consumed refined sugar and bread while taking in too few antioxidants and an insufficient supply of supplements. He was probably low in magnesium and definitely low in omega-3 oils while over indulging in omega-6 fats. Then, to top it all off, his cancer occurred on the side of his head that Phil used to talk on his cell phone, near his left ear.

Other symptoms also made life problematic. Phil suffered from high blood pressure, acid reflux, post-nasal drip, heart arrhythmias, intestinal cramping and bloating, kidney stones, occasional sharp instantaneous headaches (lasting one second), a constant mental fog, almost daily headaches lasting hours, a fungal infection on his big toe, and constant neck and back strain.

On top of all this, we shouldn't be surprised to hear that he was always tired. Fortunately, the body usually does a fantastic job of healing itself from all the insults we inflict on it. However, there may also come a time when the body becomes overwhelmed and succumbs to the bombardment of adverse conditions in one way or another.

The desmoplastic melanoma was the result of having mistreated his body—albeit unwittingly. There was a point during diagnosis and treatment when Phil did not know whether he would live long or die soon. With that uncertainty weighing on him, he went forward with picking out a burial crypt and even composing his own last words to be read during the funeral. The unknowing was scary but aroused his full attention.

DON'T LIVE PRECARIOUSLY LIKE PHIL . . . Please!!! Now that we know what Phil did wrong, let's learn from his errors. We all have the means to correct those mistakes. Proper protocols of diet, supplements, and exercise subsequently have come to save Phil's life. If his/my lifestyle had not changed, I wouldn't be here to tell the story. That is the reason for writing this book—to pass on this knowledge to help you achieve better health. Whether you follow some, most, or all of the suggested regimens, you will benefit to the degree you choose. I predict that the more you follow the recommendations, the healthier you will be. I know it worked to transform Phil into the man I am today with a healthy body, happy life; I'm a new man with purpose.

Writing this book during many different phases of surgery and treatment gave me a different perspective on life. I appreciate the love of God, family, and friends now more than ever. Life is a blessing; live it and share it now. Appreciate and love your spouse/partner, kids, parents, family, and friends.

I thank God he gave me the wisdom to learn about the things that have been growing on this earth from the time of Adam and Eve in the Garden of Eden, which was the means to nourish and heal the human body naturally. All of my previous symptoms are gone, and I FEEL GREAT!!! This may be the closest thing to the fountain of youth—the Garden of Eden lifestyle and diet, utilizing God's pharmacy of phytonutrients and supplements. To this day, I do not take or need any prescription drugs. I may be approaching 60, but my body and mind feel like I am in my mid-30's.

To say that I have studied and learned a lot about nutrients, diet, and exercise is an understatement. Ask anyone you know who has had cancer or a life changing illness. They will say they have become avid readers and tireless researchers. Why? Because nobody will have as genuine an interest in health as the afflicted person who needs it the most: necessity compels passion and devotion to learn how to help oneself.

Just for a moment, let me ask that you pretend that you have cancer—though please know I pray that you do not now have it and will not have it in the future! In this scenario, imagine that you must do everything in your power to treat the illness. With this hope in mind, I offer this book so you never have to hear those terrifying words, "YOU HAVE CANCER."

HEALTHY BODY, HAPPY LIFE

Utilizing the exercise techniques above, I have finally been able to obtain muscle tone and even build muscle efficiently despite enduring cancer and its treatment for five years. I look and feel better now in my late 50's than I did in my 20's. The constant neck and back strain are gone as the muscles I've toned keep the vertebrae in place—no need to visit the chiropractor any longer. On top of that, I have more energy and a renewed passion for life. Taking the supplements at the recommended maintenance level has fortified my heart, which does not feel like it is laboring to contract and beats much more smoothly and quietly now—like a well-oiled machine. Neither have I had any arrhythmic episodes. It just "feels" so much better, and I attribute this improved health to the supplements, diet, and exercise that I share here with you.

My wife and I recently went on a trip to Europe with 39 other friends of a special group that we belong. Most of the fellow travelers got sick with a cold or flu bug. My wife was concerned that we too would get sick. I looked at her and told her that because we practice what is preached in this book, we will not get sick. This proved true—but not to my amazement—and we enjoyed every day on vacation while others spent time in their room missing the sites.

You too can put the power of God's pharmacy to work, along with nutritious organic foods and beneficial exercise routines, to LOOK and FEEL healthier. Your future awaits! Put forth the effort now, and reap the rewards for the rest of your life.

References

Bhagavathi A. Narayanan, Otto Geoffrey, Mark C. Willingham; "Expression and its possible role in G1 arrest and apoptosis in ellagic acid treated cancer cells."; Cancer Letters; Mar 1, 1999: volume 136, issue 2, pages 215-221.

http://assets.aarp.org/rgcenter/health/rx_midlife_plus.pdf; January 2005.

http://www.aarp.org/content/dam/aarp/ppi/2014-11/rx-price-watch-report-AARP-ppi-health.pdf; Rx Price Watch Report November 2014.

http://www.chcf.org/publications/2014/07/health-care-costs-101.

http://www.commonwealthfund.org/usr_doc/856_Davis_hlt_productivity_USworkers.pdf.

YouTube videos on various exercises.

CHAPTER SEVEN
A Look At Common Diseases

When in doubt, use nutrition first.

Linus Pauling (1901-1994)
Winner of two (unshared) Nobel Prizes:
"Optimum nutrition is the medicine of tomorrow."

ALLOW ME TO share with you an encore to the work carefully laid out and explained in detail above. Chapter Six closed with words of hope and encouragement to set you on a path to healthy living. However, I would be remiss if I did not also follow up with a list of common illnesses and how best to apply the basic protocols plus specific key enhancements to mitigate those ailments. This chapter focuses on the most common diseases that Americans—and increasingly, others in the most advanced industrialized countries of the world—suffer.

Recall that inflammation is central to disease processes. The causes of chronic inflammation are free radicals, lipid peroxidation, persistent microbial infections, visceral fat producing inflammatory cytokines, AGE's, radiation exposure, and brain excitotoxins.

The most important weapon we have against causes of chronic inflammation is our diet—it can provide healthy beneficial nutrients, or it can be loaded with harmful and cancer-causing agents. The modern diet is 20 times more inflammatory than the "hunter-gatherer" type of diet. Curbing and eliminating inflammation is critical to preventing many illnesses, especially cancer.

We need a healthy diet that includes antioxidants and omega-3 fats, reduces refined sugar and glutamates, and avoids carrageenan. Supplementation is also crucial. Probiotics and vitamin D3 help boost the immune system. Many of the supplements outlined above help prevent inflammation and are even more effective when combined with a nutritious diet and regular exercise.

Instead, we bombard ourselves with harmful pesticides, pollution, GMO's, processed foods, omega-6 fats, glutamate flavor enhancers (which feed cancer by stimulating its growth and spread), and consume excessive amounts of refined sugar.

We have seen the common cause of disease—chronic inflammation. We have addressed the basic means of prevention and methods to obtain and maintain a healthy, lean body: diet, supplements, exercise, proper sleep, and avoiding harmful activities.

It is better to begin these preventive measures now, before the onset of chronic inflammation that precedes debilitating or deadly disease. *If we are too late for prevention, this chapter will offer vital information about some of the more common diseases and the regimen required to diminish, or cure, the ailment.*

When presented with a disease, we need to go beyond the baseline measures for prevention and get the body into healing mode. This requires doses of supplements higher than usual maintenance levels to combat the ailment. However, please keep in mind the recommended dosages on the manufacturers' label that denote safe levels and always adhere to their recommendations.

Please note that, depending on the brand you buy—as opposed to the brands listed in this book—the dosages suggested may be slightly different from the dosage available of your chosen brand of supplement. This is fine. Just get as close as possible to the doses recommended here for each disease while staying within stated safe limits.

Cancer

ACCORDING TO THE American Cancer Society, in 2015 there were 1.6 million new cancer diagnoses and almost 600,000 deaths. Cancer is the second leading cause of death in the U.S., second only to heart disease.

This has not always been the case. Cancer was rare in the ancient world—it is a modern, man-caused disease. Cancer rates are growing faster in the most advanced industrialized nations compared to levels in so-called third world countries. We have seen why this is true: pollution, industrial chemicals, poor diet, and harmful lifestyles, which are the reasons people suffer cancers' fate.

The good news is that while we may not be able to alter the larger conditions of environmental degradation that so negatively affect us, at least we can take control of our own lives and make changes that matter to our health. It is my firm belief that 90 percent of all cancers are preventable if we take the time to adhere to the Garden of Eden Lifestyle and diet.

Unfortunately, the World Health Organization (WHO) estimates in their 2014 World Cancer Report that cancer rates will rise by 57 percent in the next two decades. In addition, the cost for treatment is already staggering. The worldwide cost in 2010 for cancer treatment was around $1.2 trillion. In 2014, the cost of cancer medicines alone reached $100 billion as reported by the Institute for Healthcare Informatics. The U.S. spent $42 billion on cancer drugs, which is almost half of the amount spent on treatment. Prevention is the key to saving lives and addressing the financial burdens that cancer causes.

So, just what is cancer? Cancer is the abnormal and uncontrolled DNA duplication, cell division, and growth of tissue. The mutated DNA causes duplication or loss of thousands of chromosomes and the associated production of enzymes that prevent the telomeres from shortening and cancer cell death (apoptosis). Thus, cancer cells do not die by programmed DNA protocols. The cancer cells grow into large masses and may send satellite cancer cells to other parts of the body (**metastasis**). Metastatic cancers have a cure rate of just 5 to 10 percent, which is why the metastasis of cancer makes long-term survival difficult if not impossible.

The original theory of the cause of cancer is damage to DNA by inheritance of defective genes (oncogenes) or carcinogens. Researchers have since discovered that chronic inflammation is the root of cancer and that the severity of cancer depends on the body's immune response. Cancer will often begin between 10 to

40 years before detection, showing up as the result of a long-ago injury or an immune deficiency.

If you block chronic inflammation, cancer rates fall dramatically, even if the causative agent is still present. *Inflammation is part of the normal wound healing process, but the immune system response to chronic inflammation also promotes cancer development and growth.* Wound healing involves mobilization of white blood cells, stimulation of cell growth, and angiogenesis—all the same processes that are essential to cancer growth. The difference in wound healing is a short-term process whereas cancer development takes much longer. Cancer cells produce inflammatory cytokines, which produces more inflammation that stimulates more immune response and even more cancer growth. The more inflammation a cancer tumor has, the worse the prognosis.

To understand how chronic inflammation is the cause, we must look at how the body initiates cellular repair after injury. The human body has millions of primitive cells called **stem cells** floating around in the interstitial spaces, ready to create more tissue cells when injury damages the organ or tissue. They are embryonic cells that have not matured yet, and create new tissue cells in times of injury. Each tissue has its own stem cell, thus liver stem cells produce more liver cells and skin stem cells more skin.

The problem arises when the stem cell's fragile DNA mutates due to chronic inflammation (i.e., chronic free radical damage). These stem cells then become **cancer stem cells** and will form cancer tumor cells specific to the tissue from which the original stem cell was derived. Thus, a mutated pancreatic stem cell leads to a pancreatic cancer stem cell. Cancer stem cells secrete inflammatory cytokines, which promote more inflammation and make the cancer more aggressive. The cancer stem cells then produce more tumor cells, which form large cancerous tumors.

Cancer tumor cells have nuclei with thousands of mutant genes that form the proteins and enzymes necessary to cause various destructive functions. These cellular malfunctions include the non-shortening of the telomeres to prevent cancer cell death, the production of cytokines to stimulate angiogenesis, and the synthesis of nagalase to inhibit GcMAF production and thus reduce the host's immune response to cancer.

Just like normal stem cells producing normal healthy tissues, cancer stem cells function to produce cancer tumors, which grow into a large mass of abnormal cells. Cancer tumors contain one to three percent cancer stem cells, of which then produce the cancer tumor cells. Without the cancer stem cell, the cancer tumor would not form. Cancer tumor cells do not produce more tumor cells. In fact, transplanted cancer *tumor* cells to another area *would not* form a new cancer tumor. However, the transplanted cancer *stem* cells *would* develop into a full-blown cancer.

One can conclude that the cancer *stem* cell plays a primary role in prevention and cure. It is the cause of the cancer tumor itself and the spread or metastasis of cancer. Modern medicine focuses on chemotherapy and radiation treatment to kill cancer, but *these protocols only destroy cancer tumor cells and not the cancer stem cells*. Have you ever heard of loved ones who were "cancer free", only to be told they have a recurrence a few years later? The therapeutic agents have killed the tumor cells so they are gone, or reduced beyond detection size. However, the one to three percent of cancer stem cells, which are microscopic and therefore undetectable by a PET scan, will remain. Then from the immune system now weakened by chemotherapy and radiation, the cancer

CHAPTER SEVEN | A LOOK AT COMMON DISEASES

stem cells will metastasize and produce more cancer tumor cells in other parts of the body.

Chemotherapy also increases inflammation that generates free radicals which promotes cancer growth. *This is why cancer is so resilient. We need to kill the cancer stem cells without harming the surrounding normal tissues while simultaneously limiting chronic inflammation in order for treatment to be effective.* A study by Yapeng Hu and Liwu Fu that concluded that *chemotherapy and radiation treatment do not kill the cancer stem cells, only the cancer tumor cells.* The authors state, "There is increasing awareness that *cancer stem cells represent a significant challenge to effective treatment of cancer as they are resistant to current clinical drugs"* (emphasis mine). See "Targeting cancer stem cells: a new therapy to cure cancer patients," in the American Journal of Cancer Research, April 28, 2012, 2 (3): 340-356.

The fuel source for cancer cells is sugar, but the cancer cells only utilize the metabolic process of glycolysis in the cytosol to create chemical energy (ATP). We looked at this process in Chapter Two. There we found that it only created four ATP energy molecules per glucose molecule rather than the far more proficient 36 ATP molecules formed by the complete aerobic metabolism of sugar in the mitochondria. This is extremely inefficient energy production and the reason 40 percent of cancer patients die from malnutrition. Cancer cells consume most of the sugar, starving the person, and steal nutrients from the rest of the body. This is why cancer patients look so thin and depleted—they have lost a lot of weight quickly while the body tries to feed the cancer cells.

Cancer tumor cells thrive on sugar, both glucose and fructose. The tumor cells use glucose for general energy, but metabolized fructose causes mitochondrial dysfunction, aids cell division, and promotes the growth and spread of cancer.

Therefore, it is imperative that one avoid excessive fructose found in fruits and especially HFCS, the high fructose corn syrup found in soda pop.

Cancer tumors prefer sugar fermentation (glycolysis) even when there is sufficient oxygen present: cancer cells promote free radical inflammation, which damages the mitochondria. This is the **Warburg Effect** as described in 1931 by Dr. Otto Warburg, a German Nobel Prize winner. Dr. Warburg postulated that cancer results from insufficient cellular respiration due to an insult to the mitochondria. Defective mitochondria, even in the presence of sufficient oxygen, are incapable of oxidizing pyruvate in the aerobic metabolic phase. This leaves cancer cells their only option—to utilize glucose fermentation (glycolysis) for cellular energy production. Thus, the driver of cancer tumors is the decrease in or lack of mitochondrial function.

Impaired mitochondrial function is at the core of cancer development. Free radical inflammatory damage will cause mitochondrial dysfunction, as will the lack of cellular oxygen. In Dr. Warburg's book, "The Prime Cause and Prevention of Cancer" he states, "The cause of cancer is no longer a mystery, we know it occurs whenever any cell is denied 60% of its oxygen requirements." Fermentation does not require oxygen. In fact, cancer cells prefer the lack of oxygen (**hypoxia**) to thrive, unlike normal cells that require oxygen for the complete and efficient metabolism of sugar.

Because of aging and many people exercising less than they should, mitochondria in this group naturally decline in number and function. However, continuing to exercise, at all ages, helps maintain healthy cellular mitochondrial metabolism. The increased blood flow and concurrent oxygenation of tissues during exercise also helps prevent cancer.

Another way to kill tumor cells is the use of hyperbaric oxygen treatment. The process exposes patients to high levels of oxygen in a pressure chamber. This drives the cellular mitochondria to function normally and prevents cancer cells' preferred energy source—fermentation. Supplementation, especially with PQQ, further promotes the building of more cellular mitochondria.

Cancer tumors have the ability to turn on hypoxia-inducible factor (HIF) which promotes the transition of normal cells into the tumor cells to utilize glycolysis and fermentation, and allows the cells to grow even without oxygen. Cancer cells can have glycolysis turned up 200 times more than normal host cells, to make up for the highly inefficient metabolism of glucose.

In lab experiments where the mutated cancer gene for HIF was blocked, the lack of HIF caused the cancer cells to stop growing. HIF turns off the mitochondrial metabolism and drives the cancer cell into fermentation mode to produce energy. The higher the level of HIF produced, the worse the cancer prognosis, and the more aggressive the cancer. *Thus, cancer prefers the lack of oxygen to thrive and illustrates why hyperbaric chambers with oxygen therapy have shown promise for cancer treatment.*

High oxygenation of tissues from HIIT (high intensity interval training) and HIST (high intensity strength training) kills cancer cells as the deep breathing increases tissue oxygen levels and turns off HIF. Limiting blood sugar and providing proper oxygenation drives the mitochondria to the full citric acid cycle and thus decreases HIF levels and lowers the risk of cancer.

The dramatic increase in sugar consumption by humans around the world over the centuries can account for some of the dramatic increases in cancer rates. In 1820, Americans ate four pounds of sugar per year (it was mostly honey). In 2015, we consumed 150 pounds of sugar per year (refined sugar, HFCS, and sucrose). Sugar promotes insulin and IGF-1 (insulin-like growth factor) which stimulates inflammation and therefore free radicals. High levels of IGF-1 indicate high risk for cancer.

Americans also eat about 200 pounds of grain annually. Grains found in bread, pastry, cake, pie, crackers, pasta, and cereal are complex carbohydrates that are broken down into simple sugars—which fuel the cancer. Altogether, from the combination of sugar and grains, we eat on average 350 pounds of sugar each year. Throwing in the high glycemic foods and HFCS, this confirms—sadly—that we are on a death spiral!

Another cause of the cancer rate increase is the excessive use of omega-6 fats. Before 1930, Americans did not use omega-6 oils for cooking and baking. They used lard and beef tallow, which were solids. After WWII, came vegetable oils, but the preferred cooking oil was a solid, because that is what they were accustomed.

So the food industry came out with a partially hydrogenated solid oil, Crisco (trans fat), and told people this "healthy fat" prevented atherosclerosis. As we now know, trans fats are extremely unhealthy. The consumption of the unhealthy fats grew from 4.5 pounds per person in 1940, to 25 pounds per person in 2000. This is clearly significant and potentially a deadly increase in consumption.

The food industry has led people to believe all foods are good for us when many actually are not. Margarine is a manufactured butter substitute that consists of polyunsaturated omega-6 oils of soy and safflower. Many margarine brands have been hydrogenated and contain trans fats, which cause cancer and heart disease. For this reason, it is better to use real butter with the saturated fats rather than margarine.

MSG (monosodium glutamate) also causes inflammation and cancer, and its use has increased dramatically, as we discussed in some detail above. Due to non-labeling and mislabeling, we do not even know if it's in our food—which means we need to assume it is present when a "suspicious" ingredient appears on the label. Cancer cells have glutamate receptors that become stimulated from foods containing glutamate. Keep in mind that glutamate is cancer fertilizer; it causes a surge in cancer growth and metastasis.

Cancer cells have the oncogene for glutaminase, an enzyme, which converts the amino acid glutamine into glutamate. This allows cancer cells to secrete glutamate, causing the tumor to invade the surrounding tissues, which results in faster growing tumors and death. Those cancer cells with the most glutamate receptors are larger cancers, have higher metastatic rates, and result in much poorer prognosis. Melanoma is one of the most deadly cancers; not only does it have more glutamate receptors, but it also secretes high levels of glutamate. Glutaminase also stimulates the activity of cancer-cell-derived nagalase, which directly inhibits the immune system by preventing macrophage production and phagocytic activity.

Clinical nagalase tests can assess the presence and severity of cancer tumors. High levels indicate numerous cancer cells. Nagalase tests performed during treatment regimens will assess the effectiveness of therapy. If the levels of nagalase diminish, the treatment therapy is successful. If the levels increase or remain the same, therapy needs to utilize other treatment modalities. This is a great way to monitor chemotherapy and radiation treatment. It provides a concrete method to assess effectiveness; and the cost of performing the test is comparable to other blood tests.

When discussing vitamin D3, we saw how GcMAF (globulin component macrophage activating factor) plays a major role to activate the body's macrophages into killing invading organisms and cancer cells. High levels of GcMAF indicate a well-functioning immune system and keep nagalase producing cells in check. GcMAF production in the body results from three possibilities: sunlight that induces its production is skin, supplementation with vitamin D3, or taken separately as a direct GcMAF therapeutic agent if the body is unable to produce sufficient quantities.

GcMAF has many important functions:

Activates macrophages – to phagocytize and destroy cancer cells.

Increases energy production at the mitochondrial level.

Inhibits angiogenesis – stops blood supply to cancer tumors.

Stimulates apoptosis – causes the suicide of cancer cells.

Turns cancer cells into healthy cells.

Reduces the metastatic potential of human cancer cells.

Improves human nerve metabolic activity.

Counters toxic effects of cadmium.

Abolishes neuropathic pain due to nerve oxidative stress.

CHAPTER SEVEN | A LOOK AT COMMON DISEASES

Increases nerve connectivity by promoting differentiation and formation of nerve ends.

It is vital that GcMAF is present to activate macrophages. As seen in the YouTube video, https://www.youtube.com/watch?v=D1WZrnCcH24, the presence of macrophages in the area of cancer does not assure cancer's destruction. First, GcMAF must activate the macrophage, and then it will destroy the cancer cells. If there is an excess of nagalase, the GcMAF activation is inhibited and the immune system proves unproductive.

The Warburg Effect showed that cancer incapacitates the mitochondria so the cancer cell must rely on fermentation for energy. GcMAF increases mitochondrial energy production—along with ubiquinol and curcumin—and shifts cellular metabolism back into normal means. Thus, cancer cells revert into healthy cells.

GcMAF inhibits angiogenesis. Any living tissue requires a blood supply to survive; thus, a growing cancer tumor deprived of a new blood supply cannot survive. In addition, if there is no blood supply, the metastatic potential decreases. *This is very important, as the main cause of cancer morbidity is due to metastasis where the cancer tumor invades other tissues.*

Other benefits of GcMAF include improvement of nerve function and reduction of neurotoxicity. This helps prevent autism and dementia. It also promotes apoptosis so cancer cells will die on their own. GcMAF does not kill cancer cells; it stimulates the immune system by activating macrophages to kill cancer cells naturally.

Vitamin C is another one of God's pharmacy, miracle-nutrients that deserves a closer look. Dr. Linus Pauling, a graduate of Oregon State University who studied chemical engineering and a two-time Nobel Laureate, proclaimed its efficacy in fighting cancer and the common cold. The RDA of vitamin C is 60 mg per day, which at this dose prevents scurvy; but Dr. Pauling advocated higher amounts for optimal therapeutic results—one gram to be taken twice a day.

Vitamin C is a potent antioxidant that protects from free radical damage. Humans do not synthesize it internally, so our diet is its only source. Foods rich in vitamin C are dark leafy green vegetables (such as kale and broccoli), berries, and citrus fruits.

Vitamin C is very beneficial and supports numerous biological functions. It is a perfect adjunct to cancer therapy; it will reduce the side effects of treatment and improve quality of life.

Take vitamin C orally on an empty stomach so excessive iron is not absorbed along with it into the blood. Do not take it with vitamin B12, as the vitamin C will degrade the B12 and make it less effective.

Oral vitamin C has limited absorption from the intestines into the blood, which results in insufficient blood levels. A new version of vitamin C, called *liposomal vitamin C*, allows for higher blood concentrations and better transport into cells. Instead of requiring the transport system to absorb vitamin C into the cell, the liposomal vitamin C that has a lipid bilayer around the ascorbic acid molecules, is able to pass directly through the cell wall due to co-solubility.

Vitamin C is also selectively cytotoxic (poisonous) to cancer cells, and thus very important to achieve high blood and cellular levels for cancer treatment. However, oral ingestion will provide a limited effective blood level. The remedy for this involves intravenous (IV) administration of vitamin C where larger doses circulate into the blood stream to induce higher cellular concentrations. Another advantage is that direct placement into the blood stream eliminates the possibility of gastrointestinal distress (diarrhea) from larger doses of vitamin C.

For adjunctive cancer treatment, IV administration of vitamin C is highly recommended. The problem is that many oncologists will not provide this additional method of treatment. An option is to seek an outside source for IV vitamin C (IVC) treatment. One source is the Riordan Clinic, found at www.RiordanClinic.org. They are a nonprofit organization of doctors that studied and have extended the work of Dr. Linus Pauling.

Typical IV vitamin C doses are 15 to 30 grams administered twice a week. Some studies have shown that humans can tolerate up to 100 grams of vitamin C daily. The goal is to increase blood and intracellular levels into a therapeutic range that causes selective destruction only to cancer cells. Vitamin C will always be a powerful antioxidant, but at these higher concentration levels, it also has a pro-oxidant effect—but only for cancer cells.

Metabolic processes in cells can explain why the cytotoxic effect of vitamin C occurs. Cancer cells have an affinity for glucose as fuel and actively transport it inside the cancer cells. An interesting phenomenon is that the molecular shape of vitamin C is very similar to that of glucose. In fact, glucose converts into vitamin C in four enzymatic steps in the liver of non-human mammals. (Humans lack the L-gulonolactone oxidase enzyme that is critical for the last step of vitamin C synthesis, which is why we need to obtain vitamin C from our diet.) Thus, cancer cells will also actively transport vitamin C within the cell, possibly due to its comparable structural shape to glucose.

Once inside the cancer cell, the large quantity of vitamin C behaves as a pro-oxidant as it interacts with the iron. Remember, iron is required for DNA replication and cell division, which is required in significant quantities to satisfy rapid cancer growth. The interaction of the pro-oxidant vitamin C with iron releases hydrogen peroxide inside the cancer cell. This causes the cancer intracellular components to lyse (be destroyed by oxidization) from the inside out. This is why hydrogen peroxide placed on skin cuts kills bacteria—it is a powerful oxidizer.

This process effectively makes high dose IV vitamin C (IVC) into a chemotherapeutic agent that is non-toxic to healthy cells. In addition, it creates positive outcomes when administered in conjunction with chemotherapy and radiation treatment. It is also relatively inexpensive compared to traditional cancer therapies that cost tens of thousands of dollars.

In general, cancer patients become fatigued, depressed, and in pain—all symptoms of scurvy (vitamin C deficiency). Cancer patients often have low blood levels of vitamin C from excessive levels absorbed into cancer cells. Thus, IV vitamin C treatment will also relieve the scurvy symptoms and the patient will have a greater sense of well-being, have less pain, have a better appetite, and report feeling less depressed. The cancer patient on vitamin C therapy will have a better quality of life.

The all-natural chemotherapeutic agent, vitamin C, greatly improves quality of life, reduces side effects from chemotherapy/radiation treatment, and does not interfere with chemotherapeutic agents or radiation treatment. So why is there such misunderstanding about its use? My radiologist told me not to take vitamin C along with the radiation treatment, thinking it would hinder results. In the end, the radiation treatment was itself not effective for my recurrent desmoplastic melanoma, and I would have been better off taking only vitamin C treatment, not the radiation.

Glen Hyland, MD, a radiation oncologist, presented a lecture at the Riordan Clinic IVC and Cancer Symposium on October 3, 2009. The presentation "IVC, Chemotherapy, and Radiation—Are They Compatible?" demonstrates not only that they are compatible, but that *they are synergistic in that the effects of IV vitamin C boost chemo and radiation treatment.*

Another therapeutic agent, curcumin, also works well with most chemotherapy drugs. It kills cancer cells via apoptosis, cannibalization, or by disrupting the DNA replication of cell division. It also reduces radiation damage from mammograms, CT, and PET scans.

Curcumin stops cancer at every stage in its process: it stops the transformation of normal stem cells into cancer stem cells, kills cancer tumor cells, and does not harm normal cells. Lastly, it disrupts the cancer signaling process so cancer cells do not metastasize or create angiogenesis.

When curcumin combines with the typical flavonoids, especially quercetin, they become even more synergistically protective against cancer. Recent research shows that curcumin and quercetin can kill cancer stem cells, or convert them back into normal stem cells, as seen by this study: Li, Y. and Zhang, T., Cancer Letters 2014 (abstract), Li, Y. et al, Clinical Cancer Research, 2010, 16; 2580-90; Li, Y. et al, Journal Nutritional Biochemistry 2011; 22; 799-806.

Borage oil, the effects of which we have previously explored, is also a powerful agent in fighting cancer. Borage oil is better than chemotherapy drugs because chemotherapy causes free radicals and lipid peroxidation in both cancer and normal cells, while the byproduct of borage oil, DGLA, only attacks cancer cells. DGLA also does not develop multidrug resistance, as is the case with other chemotherapeutic agents, so it performs well alone or even with chemotherapeutic agents.

Protocols for Cancer

TRADITIONAL WESTERN MEDICINE treatment of cancer involves surgery, chemotherapy, and radiation. Many small cancers that have not metastasized respond well by surgical removal. The larger cancers that have metastasized require treatment that is more intensive. We have seen how cancer stem cells do not respond to chemotherapy and radiation. Therefore, as proven by studies, we must increase supplementation of specific nutrients, which kill cancer stem cells. This is especially true for borage oil (GLA), quercetin, and curcumin.

We have seen that diet, exercise, avoidance of proximity and/or intake of hazardous chemicals, and supplementation are beneficial methods to prevent cancer. We examined the basic supplement regimen for preventative health, but enhancement of the supplementation protocols to treat cancer must go beyond basic maintenance levels.

As a basic review, eat a healthy diet without refined sugar, MSG, omega-6 fats, red meat (high in iron), and high glycemic carbohydrates. The vegetables/fruits smoothie mix provides over 5,000 phytonutrients and ellagic acid—a known cancer fighter. Instead of one vegetables/fruits smoothie per day, I would consume the smoothie for breakfast and dinner. For Lunch, eat a sensible diet; chicken and fish is a good source of protein. Blueberries (a powerful antioxidant and lower in fructose) and nuts (omega-3 fats) make good snacks to keep your energy levels higher. It is a shame, but many oncology healthcare providers tell cancer patients to eat whatever they want; just keep the weight on—even if it is full of sugar—argh!

Limit carbohydrate consumption by avoiding baked goods and processed foods, which have added refined sugar. Fructose, which is in fruits and soda pop (HFCS), is also a harmful sugar that we must decide to reduce in our diet. The suggested intake of fructose should be limited to 25 grams per day for healthy people and 15 grams per day for those with cancer. See Appendix D for a table listing the amount of fructose in various fruits. Using Stevia is a good natural way to provide sweetness to foods without experiencing any detrimental side effects.

The ketogenic diet starves cancer cells of sugar while providing medium-chained triglycerides as the fuel source for brain and other tissues. This prevents the cancer cells from creating cellular energy while allowing the healthy cells to survive. Insulin and leptin resistance is very common in cancer patients and explains why those with diabetes have a higher risk of cancer and vice-versa. The ketogenic diet benefits diabetics as well.

Maintain exercise to the extent possible as it provides oxygenation of all body tissues and releases Human Growth Hormone. During some phases of treatment, exercise may be limited to just walking due to fatigue, but that's still better than doing nothing at all. It goes without saying that cessation of smoking, avoiding second-hand smoke, and refraining from drinking alcohol will promote healing, and fights cancer.

The best arsenal we have at our disposal is God's pharmacy—this was a gift from our creator to prevent and heal cancer. Vegetables and fruits, with their healing phytonutrients, have been around since the beginning of human history. Which would you trust more—divinely created vegetables and fruits with their corresponding nutrients that are healthy and safe without side effects?

Alternatively, perhaps, synthetic chemotherapeutic poisons that were recently formulated and haven't been fully tested; but are known to kill normal healthy cells and are hastily put on the market to satisfy corporate greed and profit? I know in which one to place my faith!

Supplement Protocols For Cancer

MAINTAIN THE STANDARD regimen for all supplements, with the following exceptions. In the presence of active cancer, in my opinion, I would increase the following supplements to improve health. This protocol increases the maintenance dosing of certain supplements to their safe maximum, in order to provide optimal supplemental efficiency to kill the cancer tumor and cancer stem cells.

The maintenance dose regimen of all other supplements remains the same.

Liposomal C (vitamin C)—take 1000 mg (two capsules) every two hours until six grams are taken. The spacing of every two hours allows for maximum sustained blood levels. Take without food, and not in association with iron or vitamin B12. For extreme cancers, consider IV vitamin C treatment and hyperbaric

CHAPTER SEVEN | A LOOK AT COMMON DISEASES

oxygen.

Vitamin D3—take 10,000 IU (two softgels) twice daily to fortify the immune system and promote the development of macrophages into cancer eating machines. Get your blood tested to assure blood vitamin D3 levels are around 90 ng/ml (nanograms per milliliter) for optimal GcMAF production. Have the test performed in the winter and during the summer. Exposure to sunlight in the summer can boost vitamin D3 levels so that less supplementation is required. Conversely, winter months would necessitate greater supplementation.

Magnesium—take 425 mg (three tablets) three times per day. It aids in over 300 metabolic processes and acts as both an antioxidant and anti-inflammatory agent. It also blocks glutamate receptors on cancer cells to reduce the growth, invasion, and spread of cancer. As you know, glutamate is a cancer fertilizer. Be sure to get your RBC (red blood cell) essential minerals test to maintain proper magnesium levels.

Beta 1,3/1,6 Glucan—take 100 mg (one capsule) once per day every day while cancer is present. It boosts cell mediated immunity by increasing the number of white blood cells that gobble up (phagocytize) cancer cells, and protects from radiation damage during mammograms, CT, and PET scans. Glucan enhances the cancer killing effects of several other bioflavonoids.

Borage Oil (GLA—gamma linolenic acid)—take 1300 mg (one softgel) twice daily. It produces free radicals and lipid peroxidation products *only within the cancer cell*, but not in normal host cells—only the cancer cells oxidize and die. Suspend the use of vitamin E and NSAID's (like ibuprofen) since they prevent borage oil from killing cancer cells.

Curcumin—take 800 mg (two softgels) three times per day. It is a powerful anti-inflammatory and kills cancer stem cells as seen in the study by Li and Zhang noted previously. Curcumin makes cancer cells susceptible to chemotherapy while protecting normal cells and promoting mitochondrial energy.

NAC (N-acetyl cysteine)—take 600 mg (one capsule) twice daily. It replenishes glutathione, an antioxidant and powerful detoxifier in the liver. Glutathione prevents cancer and reduces tumor growth, invasion, and metastasis. NAC can interfere with some chemotherapy drugs used during active cancer treatment; so only take NAC during non-chemotherapy periods.

PQQ (pyrroloquinoline quinone) —take 10 mg (one capsule) twice daily. It promotes the creation of more cellular mitochondria. This obstructs cancer stem cell formation, which would otherwise occur due to mitochondrial diminished function or total failure.

Quercetin with Bromelain—take 1000 mg (four capsules) three times per day. Along with curcumin, it too is a powerful anti-inflammatory and kills cancer stem cells. It also prevents angiogenesis and increases mitochondrial energy.

Ubiquinol—take 100 mg (one softgel) twice daily. The antioxidant action of ubiquinol is one of the most important functions in cellular biology as it is an essential component of the mitochondrial electron transport chain process of the citric acid cycle. Here, it transfers electrons during the synthesis of ATP in creating chemical energy. Without ubiquinol, normal host cells would not manufacture energy and would die or convert into cancer cells.

Conclusion

REMEMBER TO BE patient. It takes decades for cancer to manifest itself and therefore takes time to reverse it. *These supplements give you the best opportunity to fight cancer while maintaining strength and quality of life.* When the threat of cancer has been eliminated, you can resume the normal body maintenance levels of the supplements.

One last recommendation about cancer: get an exam from a dermatologist now. Melanoma is very deadly and its best if found early for ideal treatment results. Prevention is always easier and less expensive than treatment. I can personally testify to this fact.

References

Reya, T; Morrison, SJ; Clarke, MF; Weissman, IL (Nov 1, 2001). "Stem cells, cancer, and cancer stem cells" *Nature* 414 (6859): 105–11. doi:10.1038/35102167. PMID 11689955.

Blaylock, R.L., Blaylock wellness report, Feb. 16 - Mar.15, 2005.

Blaylock, R.L., Blaylock wellness report, October 2008.

O'connor, M. L., Et. Al., Cancer Lett 2014; 344: 180-7.

http://articles.mercola.com/sites/articles/archive/2015/11/23/vitamin-c-curative-power.aspx.

http://orthomolecular.org/library/jom/2008/pdf/2008-v23n04-p183.pdf.

articles.mercola.com/sites/articles/archive/2014/03/02/curcumin-benefits.aspx?e_cid=1stBestOfNL_art_5&et_cid=DM89376&et_rid=1380673353.

Greenmedinfo.com, Curcumin.

Dementia

DEMENTIA IS THE third leading cause of death, after heart disease and cancer. Also known as senility, it includes a broad category of brain diseases that cause gradual loss of one's ability to think and remember, in addition to loss of emotions and motor skills. Dementia will affect the brain in different areas that lead to a particular diagnosis, some of which are Alzheimer's, Parkinson's, autism, or ALS (amyotrophic lateral sclerosis—or Lou Gehrig's disease). Dementia symptoms can overlap when numerous brain areas are affected.

Alzheimer's is the most common type of dementia and affects the hippocampus—the center for learning and memory. This is why Alzheimer's patients will not remember their relatives, but will retain speech skills since language functions in the left-brain hemisphere. Parkinson's affects the substantia nigra—the brain component that controls voluntary muscle movement. This accounts for the uncontrolled shaking noticed in these patients.

What is the cause of dementia? Two related processes cause neurological disorders: chronic cranial inflammation and excitotoxicity. Both stimulate overactivity of the microglia, which releases free radicals (peroxynitrite, a powerful toxin) and immune-related cytokines such as TNF alpha (tumor necrosis factor alpha). TNF alpha affects receptors on neurons that cause their destruction and leads to the build-up of amyloid-beta protein, a neural plaque that hinders nerve transmission and brain function, causing dementia. As the disease progresses, the inflammation intensifies and the condition accelerates.

There are many causes of brain inflammation and excitotoxicity. These include excessive glutamate, sugar, mercury,

Aluminum, lead, systemic fluoride, pesticides, industrial/household chemicals, vaccine adjuvants, aspartame, viruses, and loss of cellular mitochondrial functions. They initiate the brain's microglial immune system.

Most damage by microglial activation is due to excitotoxicity in response to extracellular glutamate. Glutamate accounts for 90 percent of neurotransmission and it regulates the other neurotransmitters: serotonin, dopamine, and acetylcholine. Glutamate can cause brain cell death in about an hour due to over stimulation of the glutamate receptors on the brain cells, which damages neurons and synapses. The reason our brain cells are not excited to death is that the nerve cells continually pump the glutamate *inside* the cell where it is harmless and functions as a neurotransmitter. Very little glutamate escapes to the outside of the cell. However, ingesting glutamate from food exposes the brain to excessive extracellular amounts of the toxic chemical.

Extracellular glutamate will break down the blood-brain barrier making it more susceptible to absorbing, and the effects of, MSG and other neurotoxins like pesticides. This will accelerate dementia.

Aspartame, the artificial sweetener, becomes glutamate during a metabolic process. Excessive consumption of this sweetener can lead to excessive glutamate conversion and the resulting inflammation. Glutamate also lowers glutathione levels, the protective antioxidant. Without antioxidant defense, neurodegenerative damage will ensue.

The excitotoxin, sugar, is a carbohydrate found in many foods. High glycemic foods with complex sugars metabolize into the simple sugar, glucose. High fructose corn syrup is also a concern. Both sugars cause free radicals and the corresponding inflammation, which stimulate the brain microglia.

Remember that the brain metabolizes most of its energy via sugar and thus creates many free radicals.

Could this be the reason that Phil got a headache when he ate too much refined sugar? The brain was telling him to stop this insult!

Another concern is the repeated cyclic rise of blood sugar levels with the corresponding cyclic rise in insulin, which can lead to insulin resistance. When this process happens in the brain, due to the brain cells' insulin resistance, it causes **Type 3 diabetes**. This is a form of diabetes that occurs only in the brain and is considered a cause for Alzheimer's disease. The chronic excessive supply of sugar occurs because it fails to absorb into the brain cells and creates inflammation. Research shows diabetics have increased risk for developing Alzheimer's disease.

The metals mercury, aluminum, and lead, plus systemic fluoride, are excitotoxins that accumulate in brain tissue. Once deposited in the tissue, it's hard to get rid of it. They have synergistic effects and cause more brain damage when associated with each other.

Mercury is extremely toxic with no known safe levels. It comes from the atmosphere (coal burning), seafood (tuna), dental silver-alloy fillings, and vaccines (see Appendix A for flu shot adjuvants).

Exposure to aluminum from eating cheese, sea-salt, black tea, soybeans, and alum in baking powder will increase aluminum blood levels. Soy is the number one source for Aluminum and, along with glutamate, makes soy a very toxic food to eat. Acidic ingredients in aluminum cans will leach aluminum into food. Citric acid (found in citrus fruits) binds Aluminum and increases

CHAPTER SEVEN | A LOOK AT COMMON DISEASES

absorption in the gastrointestinal (GI) tract—so do not add lemon slices to black tea (it is fine in white or green tea). Vaccines also have aluminum additives.

Aluminum also interferes with mitochondrial energy production causing brain cells to have less energy, which increases sensitivity to excitotoxicity. Aluminum competes with magnesium, resulting in less ATP energy production.

Aluminum also forms the salt of aluminum glutamate, which is readily absorbed by the GI tract and blood-brain barrier. Then the glutamate activates microglia receptors and stimulates the immune response to increase inflammation. Aluminum can also concentrate in the myelin sheath of neural pathways and cause the degenerative disease called multiple sclerosis.

Lead use has greatly diminished, especially since its removal from gasoline and paint many years ago. However, some manufacturing still use it today. Fortunately, the risk for lead exposure is low.

Fluoride is the salt form of fluorine and causes dementia as well as cancer and thyroid suppression. Systemic fluoride accumulates in brain tissues until excitotoxic levels cause inflammation and dementia. It is synergistic with and potentiates aluminum to create more brain cell damage. Systemic fluoride accumulates in the long bones and can cause cancer—osteosarcoma. Fluoride uptake can weaken the cortical bone plate (outer bone cover) resulting in more prevalent hip fractures (as seen in the elderly).

The thyroid accumulates systemic fluoride and inhibits the thyroid from using iodine to make the thyroid hormone. This causes thyroid suppression or hypothyroidism, which can affect metabolism and energy. Hypothyroidism increases with age and can affect as many as 60 percent of the population.

As a side note, pregnant moms should not use fluoride supplementation as it passes through the placenta and accumulates in the fetal thyroid gland—not to mention the brain. For these reasons, I do not prescribe fluoride tablets for ingestion by my dental patients. The benefit of fluoride on teeth is from direct contact with the tooth surface; systemic fluoride does not provide this direct contact. In addition, some supplement gelatin capsules of animal-source origin may contain fluoride. Instead, use vegan or vegetable capsules.

Vaccines have many cytotoxic adjuvants that promote dementia. Remember they are cumulative and cytotoxic. See Appendix A for a complete list.

With all the glutamate, artificial sweeteners, refined sugar, mercury, Aluminum, systemic fluoride, pesticides, chemicals, viruses, and vaccines invading our bodies, is there any doubt about why dementia is so prevalent, and becoming more so by the day? Alzheimer's is the sixth leading cause of death.

Protocols for Dementia

AS WITH ANY form of treatment, start by eliminating foods that promote the problem–those, which stimulate brain inflammation. Stay away from all soy products (high in MSG and aluminum), glutamate (flavorings), processed meats (nitrates/nitrites), and avoid eating excessive red meat (which is high in iron). In addition, avoid refined sugar (especially HFCS and processed white bread), tuna fish (mercury), partially hydrogenated oils (trans

CHAPTER SEVEN | A LOOK AT COMMON DISEASES

fats), omega-6 oils, and fluoridated water. Also, avoid food wrapped in aluminum and food in tin cans, especially tomatoes. The acids from tomatoes along with the bisphenol A (BPA) from the tin-can plastic lining generate toxins. The good news is that some food manufacturers are aware of the problem with BPA and no longer put the toxic BPA lining in the tin can. The tin-can front labels often reflects this practice—support these product manufacturers, as they are concerned about your health.

Supplement Protocols for Dementia

IT IS IMPORTANT to follow the general supplement maintenance protocols for basic health protection. Other, more dementia-protective supplements should be increased in dosage. The following list includes increases in dosage of supplements that I would personally recommend for a family member or myself when confronted with the diagnosis of dementia.

Liposomal C (vitamin C)—take 1000 mg (two capsules) every two hours for a total of six per day. Vitamin C protects the brain and can effectively remove aluminum from the body. The brain has the highest concentration of vitamin C levels, especially the hippocampus (the memory/learning center) and the amygdala (the center that processes complex pain and fear reactions). These two areas just happen to be the target of Alzheimer's. *Is there a coincidence that low levels of vitamin C occur in patients with Alzheimer's disease?*

Alzheimer's patients that have lower levels of vitamin C experience faster cognitive decline. Moreover, those with damage to the blood-brain barrier developed Alzheimer's more quickly—because the damage allows dietary glutamate to enter the brain space. Vitamin C maintains the blood-brain barrier and protects the brain. Vitamin C also reduces a type of beta amyloid plaque, called abeta oligomers, found in Alzheimer's patients.

Parkinson's disease is due to a lack of dopamine. Vitamin C stimulates the brain's manufacture of dopamine and thus may help prevent this form of dementia. Both vitamin C and vitamin E are important to relieve the brain's oxidative stress, but vitamin C is more important for brain protection.

In elderly people, the vitamin C transport mechanism to get vitamin C into the hippocampus is less effective. Increasing oral vitamin C is of no use. Since the brain is 60 percent fat, a fat-soluble form of vitamin C is required. Liposomal vitamin C is fat-soluble and absorbs directly into the cells where needed and provides protection.

Vitamin D3—take 10,000 IU (two softgels) twice daily. It improves insulin levels, lowers blood sugar, and improves insulin resistance. Thus, it reduces the chance of developing Type 3 diabetes and the resulting inflammation. Vitamin D3 also reduces brain inflammation by modulating microglia activity, presumably by the promotion of GcMAF.

Get your blood tested to assure the blood vitamin D3 levels are around 90 ng/ml (nanograms per milliliter), for optimal GcMAF production. Have the test performed in the winter and during the summer. Exposure to sunlight in the summer can boost vitamin D3 levels so that less supplementation is required. Conversely, winter months would necessitate increased supplementation.

Magnesium—take 425 mg (three tablets) three times daily. It binds to glutamate receptors and decreases glutamate's toxicity by inhibiting stimulation of the inflammatory immune TNF-alpha cytokine. Thus, it decreases microglia activation and damage. Magnesium also chelates (binds to) mercury and removes it from the brain to reduce excitotoxicity.

Acetyl-l-carnitine—take 500 mg (one capsule) twice daily. It repairs mitochondria and restores energy levels. Acetyl-L-carnitine also improves nerve function and protects against excitotoxicity. Do not take this with anti-depressants; the result could over stimulate brain cells.

Curcumin—take 400 mg (one softgel) three times per day. It increases mitochondrial energy and reduces microglial activation from its anti-inflammatory and antioxidant properties. This protects the brain from beta-amyloid plaques. It also improves insulin resistance, promotes uptake of sugar into muscle cells, and decreases Type 3 diabetes risk.

DHA (Docosahexaenoic acid)—take 560 mg (two softgels) three times daily with food. It decreases glutamate excitotoxicity by decreasing brain inflammation, and it inhibits a microglia response.

Grape seed extract—take 100 mg (one capsule) two times daily. It is a powerful antioxidant and anti-inflammatory that provides brain protection from glutamate.

NAC (N-acetyl-cysteine)—take 600 mg (one capsule) twice daily. It increases glutathione levels (the main cellular antioxidant, especially for liver detoxification) that chelates mercury to rid it from the brain.

PQQ (pyrroloquinoline quinone)—take 10 mg (one capsule) twice daily. It maintains and synthesizes more cellular mitochondria. This attribute helps decrease Type 3 diabetes and promotes glucose consumption. PQQ is also an antioxidant, which relieves oxidative stress and the resultant inflammation.

Quercetin with Bromelain—take 500 mg (two capsules) three times daily. The anti-inflammatory and antioxidant qualities increase mitochondrial energy and reduce microglial activation. Along with curcumin, this protects the brain from beta-amyloid plaques, improves insulin resistance, promotes uptake of sugar into muscle cells, and decreases Type 3 diabetes risk.

Conclusion

IN ADDITION TO the supplements, replacement of sugar by MCT oil, coconut oil, and olive oil, transforms the energy source for the brain into ketones. We have seen how the brain can use this alternate energy source. It is beneficial in preventing dementia as well as cancer. We will see shortly that a ketogenic diet also reduces metabolic syndrome (heart disease, diabetes, and obesity).

To prevent dementia, it is also important to challenge your mind daily. Mental stimulation by learning something new or engaging the mind in deep-thought games is associated with decreased risk. The consensus among researchers is that the active mind repairs and develops new neural pathways, thus making the mind less susceptible to beta-amyloid plaque and dementia.

References

https://www.nlm.nih.gov/medlineplus/ency/article/000739.htm.

Blaylock, R.L., Blaylock wellness report, May 2004.

http://www.niddk.nih.gov/health-information/health-topics/Diabetes/hypoglycemia/Pages/index.aspx.

Blaylock, R.L., Blaylock wellness report, Sept 2004.

Autoimmune Disorders

AUTOIMMUNE DISEASES RESULT from the body's immune system mistakenly attacking its own body tissues. This provokes inflammation and the cascade response that destroys tissues and causes organ dysfunction. There are many theories about the causes of autoimmunity, but they are associated with genetic factors. The good news is that the incidence rate in our population is low; the bad news is that autoimmune disorders are often chronic, incapacitating, and at times deadly. Statistics show autoimmune disorders to be the tenth leading cause of death among American women up to the age of 65. Autoimmune disorders cause over 80 diseases.

This partial list shows the tissue or organ affected, followed by the particular, more common disorders:

Heart: subacute bacterial endocarditis

Skin: alopecia, lichen planus, psoriasis

Salivary Glands: Sjogren's syndrome

Digestive System: celiac disease, Crohn's disease, ulcerative colitis

Blood: pernicious anemia, thrombocytopenia

Connective Tissue: rheumatic fever, rheumatoid arthritis

Muscle: fibromyalgia, myasthenia gravis

Nervous System: Guillain-Barre syndrome, multiple sclerosis, restless leg syndrome

Eyes: Grave's disease

Ears: Meniere's disease

Vascular System: lupus vasculitis

Kidney: lupus nephritis

Adrenal Gland: Addison's disease

Pancreas: diabetes mellitus Type 1

As we can see, many tissues and organs are affected. The common treatment for autoimmunity includes immunosuppression medications that decrease the immune response and lessen the autoimmune effects. However, at what cost? With systemic medications that affect the entire body, there will be areas of the body where immune suppression will be detrimental–especially those areas of cancer that progress unabated. There are natural supplements and strategies that lessen the effects of autoimmune disorders. Let's look at two of them and their remedies.

Multiple Sclerosis

THIS IMMUNE-MEDIATED disease is the one that most commonly affects the central nervous system. It damages the insulating layer (myelin sheath) around the nerve cells in the brain and spinal cord. The name multiple sclerosis (MS) refers to the many sclerae (scars or lesions) that form on the nerve sheath in the brain or spinal cord. The damage disrupts nerve conduction, and depending upon the location of scarred nerve tissue, presents various signs and symptoms, which aid in the diagnosis. These

CHAPTER SEVEN | A LOOK AT COMMON DISEASES

patients usually exhibit visual, motor, and sensory problems, along with problems of the auto-regulated functions like breathing, heart rate, urination, and digestion.

The most noticeable sign is loss of motor control that leads to muscle weakness, muscle spasms, difficulty moving, and especially difficulty with coordination and balance. Other noticeable signs are trouble with speech and straining to swallow. These people are often tired and experience acute or chronic pain.

MS usually begins from age 20 to 50. It also affects twice as many women as men. The cause of nerve damage appears to be genetic and environmental factors such as infections that provoke the microglial immune system to attack the myelin sheath.

There is no known cure, and medications have limited results with harsh side effects.

Prednisone, a steroid drug, is a common treatment for MS. However, long-term steroid use has proven to produce its own debilitating effects. The long-term prognosis is hard to predict, but women have better overall outcomes with this drug. The overall life expectancy is 5 to 10 years shorter than the unaffected.

Even though a cure is not available, vitamin D3 shows promise to help repair myelin damage. As reported by a University of Cambridge study,

> *"By adding vitamin D to brain stem cells where the proteins were present, they found the production rate of oligodendrocytes (myelin making cells) increased by 80 percent. When they blocked the vitamin D receptor to stop it from working, the RXR gamma protein alone was unable to stimulate the production of oligodendrocytes."*

This study can be viewed at http://www.dddmag.com/news/2015/12/vitamin-d-could-repair-nerve-damage-ms-study-suggests.

Statistics show that people with MS have a vitamin D3 deficiency. We have seen how sunlight can boost D3 levels and that scientists have explored safe ways to do this. Get tested to make sure you aren't deficient.

Dementia-causing diseases like Parkinson's and Alzheimer's are associated with brain shrinkage, a result of poor functioning mitochondria. MS patients also show signs of brain shrinkage, which could be the effect of dysfunctional mitochondria as well. This could explain why MS patients are easily fatigued. Ways to promote mitochondria growth are consuming more omega-3 fats and less omega-6 fats, while taking ubiquinol (the reduced form of CoQ10) and PQQ (pyrroloquinoline quinone).

Other factors can affect multiple sclerosis. Mercury, MSG, and aspartame cause excitotoxicity and mimic autoimmune disorders. Nicotine (even from patches) is a powerful immune suppressant, which makes people more prone to infection. The immune-suppression can increase the risk of developing an autoimmune disorder, especially for people who have been vaccinated. These are more good reasons to avoid mercury, MSG, sugar substitutes, smoking, and vaccines.

Supplement Protocols For Multiple Sclerosis

CONTINUE THE SUPPLEMENTS for routine maintenance as described in Chapter Six. However, I recommend increasing the dosage of the following supplements.

Vitamin D3—take 10,000 IU (two softgels) twice daily. It reduces brain inflammation by modulating microglia activity and promotes regeneration of the myelin protective sheath around nerves.

Magnesium—take 425 mg (three tablets) three times daily. It binds to glutamate receptors and decreases glutamate's toxicity. Magnesium decreases microglia activation and nerve damage. It also chelates (binds to) mercury and removes it from the brain to reduce excitotoxicity.

Curcumin—take 400 mg (one softgel) three times daily. This powerful anti-inflammatory and antioxidant agent increases mitochondrial energy and reduces brain microglial activation.

DHA (Docosahexaenoic acid)—take 560 mg (two softgels) three times daily with food. It decreases glutamate excitotoxicity by decreasing brain inflammation and inhibits the microglia response.

PQQ (pyrroloquinoline quinone)—take 10 mg (one capsule) twice daily. It maintains and synthesizes more cellular mitochondria. PQQ is also an antioxidant, which relieves oxidative stress and the resultant inflammation. It helps provide energy to nerve cells for repair and lessens patient fatigue.

Quercetin with Bromelain—take 500 mg (two capsules) three times daily. This is another powerful anti-inflammatory and antioxidant agent, acting to increase mitochondrial energy and reduce brain microglial activation.

Rheumatoid Arthritis

RHEUMATOID ARTHRITIS (RA) IS an autoimmune disorder

caused by genetic and environmental factors. The body attacks its own joints, resulting in inflammation and enlargement of the joint capsule. It causes pain, stiffness, and can be quite crippling, especially in the hands. It has a slow onset but progressively worsens in the chronic state.

Rheumatoid arthritis affects less than 1 percent of adults, with the onset occurring during middle age. Chronic effects of RA can be fatal as it manifests in other tissues and organs such as lungs, kidneys, and the heart, with a lifespan reduced by 3 to 12 years. RA victims encounter twice the risk for heart disease, irrespective of other metabolic syndrome risk factors.

Pain medications and steroids (prednisone) may relieve symptoms, while some anti-rheumatic drugs may slow its progression, but they also have adverse side effects. Reports show methotrexate, an anti-rheumatic drug, to cause fibrosis of the lungs—scarring and thickening that makes it harder to breathe. Side effects include nausea, vomiting, and abdominal pain. Fifteen percent of patients develop increased liver enzymes requiring liver biopsies.

Despite the debilitation from RA and the harmful medication side effects, dietary measures can provide great benefit. Chronic inflammation plays a prominent role in the disease process, aided by the dietary consumption of fructose and other sugars. Reduction of all sugars, especially HFCS, will reduce inflammation and RA progression. See Appendix D, which lists the amount of fructose in fruits.

In the American Journal of Clinical Nutrition, 2014, researchers found that RA flourishes from soda pop consumption. They determined that women who drank one or more sodas per day had a 63 percent increased chance of having RA, compared to women who drank less than one can of soda per month, or none at all. This again shows the importance of limiting HFCS in soda pop and fructose in general. The study can be found on the website for the July 16, 2014 publication located in the reference section. Since women suffer RA 2.5 times more frequently than men, this study focused on the female gender.

Omega-3 fats consumption goes a long way to reduce lipid peroxidation and inflammation. These healthy fats include olive oil, avocados, coconut oil, DHA, and even GLA (gamma linolenic acid). GLA may reduce pain and stiffness in the affected joints, as well as eating organic whole foods, which effectively reduce inflammation as well.

The main goal with diet is to prevent inflammation and promote cellular health by assisting the mitochondria. Proper functioning mitochondria help reduce autoimmune inflammation. We previously examined nutritious foods and know to avoid processed and GMO food. In addition, probiotics are paramount to maintaining a healthy gut flora that boosts the immune system.

As with MS patients, those suffering from RA also find their vitamin D3 levels are generally too low. Vitamin D3 helps regulate the immune system to fight infections and inflammation. Thus, it is important to test vitamin D3 levels and maintain therapeutic concentrations.

Curcumin is a potent anti-inflammatory agent, effective against acute and chronic pain. It inhibits inflammatory enzymes and blocks inflammation pathways. A 2012 study revealed that curcumin was more effective in alleviating RA symptoms than some NSAIDs (non-steroidal anti-inflammatory drugs). It also showed improvement in reducing its progression.

Supplement Protocols For Rheumatoid Arthritis

CONTINUE THE BASIC maintenance protocols, but in treating RA, I recommend revised dosages for the following supplements as noted:

Vitamin D3—take 10,000 IU (two softgels) twice daily. It reduces inflammation and assists the immune system in fighting infection. Get tested to maintain therapeutic levels.

Magnesium—take 425 mg (three tablets) three times daily. This essential element aids in over 300 biological processes; it acts as both an anti-inflammatory and antioxidant agent.

Borage Oil (GLA—gamma linolenic acid)—take 1300 mg (one softgel) twice daily. It helps reduce inflammation and joint pain.

Curcumin—take 400 mg (one softgel) three times daily. This powerful anti-inflammatory and antioxidant agent increases mitochondrial energy and reduces inflammation.

DHA (Docosahexaenoic acid)—take 560 mg (two softgels) three times daily with food. It decreases inflammation and helps reduce joint pain.

PQQ (pyrroloquinoline quinone)—take 10 mg (one capsule) twice daily. It maintains and synthesizes more cellular mitochondria. PQQ is also an antioxidant, which relieves oxidative stress and the resultant inflammation.

Quercetin with Bromelain—take 500 mg (two capsules) three times daily. Along with curcumin, both are powerful anti-inflammatory and antioxidant agents that increase mitochondrial

CHAPTER SEVEN | A LOOK AT COMMON DISEASES

energy and reduce inflammation.

References

Cotsapas C, Hafler DA (2013). "Immune-mediated disease genetics: the shared basis of pathogenesis". Trends in Immunology 34 (1): 22–6. doi:10.1016 / j.it.2012.09.001. PMID 23031829.

Walsh, SJ; Rau, LM (September 2000). "Autoimmune diseases: a leading cause of death among young and middle-aged women in the United States.". American Journal of Public Health 90 (9): 1463–6. doi:10.2105 / ajph.90.9.1463. PMC 1447637.PMID 10983209.

Compston A, Coles A (October 2008). "Multiple sclerosis" . Lancet 372 (9648): 1502–17. doi:10.1016/S0140-6736(08)61620-7.PMID 18970977.

http://jcb.rupress.org/content/211/5/936.1.full.

http://www.dddmag.com/news/2015/12/vitamin-d-could-repair-nerve-damage-ms-study-suggests.

http://www.ncbi.nlm.nih.gov/pubmed/2087010.

Singh, JA; Wells, GA; Christensen, R; Tanjong Ghogomu, E; Maxwell, L; Macdonald, JK; Filippini, G; Skoetz, N; Francis, D; Lopes, LC; Guyatt, GH; Schmitt, J; La Mantia, L; Weberschock, T; Roos, JF; Siebert, H; Hershan, S; Lunn, MP; Tugwell, P; Buchbinder, R (16 February 2011). "Adverse effects of biologics: a network meta-analysis and Cochrane overview.". *The Cochrane database of systematic reviews* (2): CD008794.doi:10.1002/14651858.CD008794.pub2. PMID 21328309.

http://articles.mercola.com/sites/articles/archive/2016/02/03/rheumatoid-arthritis-medications.aspx?e_cid=20160203Z1_DNL_art_1&utm_source=dnl&utm_medium=email&utm_content=art1&utm_campaign=20160203Z1&et_cid=DM96832&et_rid=1342307222.

American Journal of Clinical Nutrition, July 16, 2014—Links RA with soda consumption.

Cardiovascular Disease

CARDIOVASCULAR DISEASE (CVD) is the number one cause of death in the United States. In 2011, nearly 800,000 people died from conditions involving the heart and blood vessels. CVD includes coronary artery disease (angina and heart attacks), strokes, high blood pressure, aneurysms, fibrillation, peripheral artery disease, and other conditions.

Coronary artery disease takes the lives of nearly 400,000 people annually and is the most common type of heart disease. It is primarily due to atherosclerosis.

Heart attacks occur in over 700,000 people per year and nearly 40 percent are recurrent. The costs of CVD are staggering. From health expenditures and lost productivity, the total is over $320 billion per year. Prevention is far less expensive, and healthier, than the cure.

Studies estimate that 90 percent of CVD is preventable. Factors that help prevent its devastating effects are nutrition, exercise, proper sleep, not smoking, and limiting alcohol use.

Studies have also shown there is a direct correlation between gum disease and heart disease. If your gums are unhealthy, bacteria get into your body through bleeding gums. The bacteria travel through the bloodstream and deposit in heart tissue and blood vessels,

CHAPTER SEVEN | A LOOK AT COMMON DISEASES

causing chronic inflammation. This is a great reason to brush and floss. In addition to saving your teeth, your heart and circulatory system will be healthier.

Most cardiovascular diseases are age dependent, and the risk increases with age.

Age	Percentage of People with CVD
20 to 30	11%
40 to 60	37%
60 to 80	71%
85 plus	85%

It is surprising these statistics are so low when you consider just what the heart does, day after day—the heart beats about 100,000 times per day, pumping 2,000 gallons of blood through 60,000 miles of blood vessels.

The underlying cause of cardiovascular disease is chronic inflammation, especially for atherosclerosis and hypertension (high blood pressure). We will look at these two types of cardiovascular diseases, plus arrhythmias, in this section and address cerebral vascular accident (CVA—stroke of brain blood vessels, which damages its nerve tissues) in the next section.

Atherosclerosis

ATHEROSCLEROSIS, OR HARDENING of the arteries, results from a build-up of plaque on the blood vessel inner wall. Plaque develops slowly over the years primarily from oxidized omega-6 fats in the blood stream. The oxidized omega-6 fats enter the wall of the blood vessel, which triggers inflammation and the immune response. The ensuing macrophages gobble up the oxidized oils and release components that make up the atherosclerotic plaque. The engorged macrophages, called foam cells, are abundant in atherosclerosis.

The blood vessel forms a fibrous cap over the plaque to protect the rest of the body from further inflammation. A stable encapsulated plaque poses no problem. However, if an unstable plaque does not fully encapsulate the inflammation, the fibrous cap can rupture into the blood vessel. This releases caustic, inflamed, oxidized oil back into the blood vessel, which contacts flowing blood. The caustic, oxidized oil triggers the blood to coagulate and forms a clot that blocks blood flow in smaller vessels downstream from the original plaque location. This process usually does not involve complete closure of the vessel, but it does restrict blood flow and reduces oxygenation of dependent tissues. The longer the restriction exists, the more it will expand and further constrict the vessel. *When the clot causes significant blockage in a heart artery, it is a myocardial infarction or heart attack. When it occurs in the arteries to brain cells, it is a stroke.*

It is important to note that *un-oxidized* oils and *un-oxidized* cholesterol cannot enter the vessel walls, will not instigate inflammation, and thus do not cause atherosclerotic plaques. To prevent oxidation of oils and cholesterol, antioxidants are critical. Remember that small, dense LDL is the most easily oxidized cholesterol and the reason it gets all the attention. Anything that produces free radicals will cause oxidation of these fats (lipid peroxidation), such as excess sugar, iron, autoimmune diseases, hazardous chemicals, toxic metals, and infections. Inflammatory bacteria found in periodontal (gum) disease, have also been found in blood vessel atherosclerotic plaques, which is why it's important to brush, floss, and get dental gum care regularly—the health of your cardiovascular system may depend on this direct connection.

Recall the study in 1950 by Dr. John Gofman who claimed triglycerides played a larger role in atherosclerosis and heart disease than cholesterol. Triglycerides levels are most affected and associated with consumption of refined sugar and high glycemic carbohydrates. High triglyceride levels are promoted by excessive sugar (and HFCS) consumption and they are converted into small dense LDL—the most oxidized cholesterol component. If you limit these dietary sugars, the triglycerides levels will be reduced, the LDL will be lower, and the HDL will be higher. Therefore, reduce your sugar intake to reduce the triglycerides and reduce risk of inflammation and atherosclerosis. This also helps to regulate insulin levels and ward off hunger.

Aging is responsible for increased atherosclerosis. The older we get the more likely it is that we will develop this unwanted plaque in our blood vessels. A study done in 2009 by Alan R. Collins looked at young and middle-aged mice, fed either a low fat, or high fat diet—no mice were fed cholesterol. They later examined the blood vessels for plaque build-up.

The middle-aged mice developed extreme atherosclerosis, especially on the high fat diet. Even low fat diets induced atherosclerosis in middle-aged mice. Since cholesterol was not present in the diet of young or middle-aged mice, researchers assumed cholesterol played a small, if any, role in development of atherosclerosis. The middle-aged mice showed higher triglyceride levels, which we noted in the cholesterol section in Chapter Two and which are the better indicator for those who will develop atherosclerosis.

Middle-aged mice had twice the free radical and lipid peroxidation products than the young mice. The difference between young and middle-aged mice was not the response to free radicals from the high fat diet, because each group would produce equal amounts of free radicals. The difference was the inability of the middle-aged mice to increase their antioxidant response to the high levels of free radicals—their antioxidant levels actually decreased due to age, which made the vessels more susceptible to free radical damage and inflammation.

By age 70, people have 10 to 15 times more free radicals than at age 35—coupled with a decrease in antioxidants that makes chronic inflammation and disease more prevalent.

The bottom-line take-home message is that older people require more abundant antioxidants than younger people do. Proper diet and supplements will accomplish this task. This means taking bioflavonoid antioxidants such as berries (blueberries, blackberries, raspberries, and strawberries), and supplements like curcumin, quercetin, Mg, NAC, ubiquinol, melatonin, aged garlic extract, and vitamins C and E. Antioxidants reduce atherosclerosis by 50 percent—which is far better than statins.

There are glutamate receptors in the blood vessel wall, and when stimulated with MSG, they will create high levels of free radicals and cause lipid peroxidation, which leads to chronic inflammation. This can last for years. Combined with older peoples' decrease in antioxidant levels, this puts them at an increased risk of atherosclerosis.

Toxic metals like mercury, lead, cadmium, iron, manganese,

and copper accelerate atherosclerosis due to the free radicals produced in the endothelial cell wall. This is another reason to avoid these metals. Green Tea Extract will reduce atherosclerosis risk by inhibiting the free radical and lipid peroxidation effects of iron in blood vessels and strengthening blood vessel walls. Green tea extract also reduces total cholesterol by reducing triglycerides and elevating HDL.

The status quo treatment for atherosclerosis has been administration of statin pharmaceuticals to decrease cholesterol levels. The problem with this regimen is two-fold. First, cholesterol is a vital biological component required by the human body to survive. Second, high triglyceride levels, not cholesterol, are to the main cause of atherosclerosis.

To control plaque build-up in arteries, it is more prudent to reduce triglyceride levels by reducing blood sugar levels—this also aids in preventing cancer, diabetes, obesity, and high blood pressure—a win, win, win, win, win situation. How awesome is that?

Cholesterol is required to make cortisol (the stress hormone) and sex hormones (estrogen, progesterone, and testosterone). It is required for the body to make vitamin D3—and we have already seen how vital D3 is in aiding the immune system to ward off cancer.

Cholesterol forms bile salts and is an antioxidant. Serotonin receptors in the brain use cholesterol for proper growth of the baby's brain, and it helps in nervous and immune system development. It promotes proper intestine function (helps prevent leaky gut syndrome), and repairs damaged cell walls.

It does not make sense to reduce this vital lipoprotein when it is a minor factor in causing atherosclerosis—especially when prescribing statins, which have numerous detrimental side effects.

Statin drug side effects include depletion of ubiquinol (CoQ10) and magnesium, which can cause heart failure and death, while impairing heart muscle mitochondria that decreases cellular energy. They cause peripheral neuropathy, or pain and crippling weakness in the limbs and joints. More side effects are reduced cognitive function with increased aggressiveness and violence, plus brain damage to the memory and learning center (hippocampus). By inhibiting the synthesis and function of vitamin K2, statins can raise your risk for atherosclerosis, heart failure, and stroke.

Statin-induced insulin resistance promotes high blood sugar levels, which promotes chronic inflammation, and heart disease. Ironically, this was the reason for the statin prescription in the first place. Insulin resistance leads to visceral fat, diabetes, heart disease, cancer, and dementia.

In addition, the decrease in cholesterol levels cause increased mortality due to less brain protection, cell wall degradation, lack of steroid synthesis, and immune suppression (reduced vitamin D3). Lower cholesterol levels also increase insomnia, anxiety and panic attacks, while decreasing libido (reduced sex hormone levels).

Statins do not lower atherosclerosis risk by reducing cholesterol; rather, they work by reducing inflammation and suppressing immunity. This is harmful in the end as chronic inflammation can develop into cancer, infections, and other diseases. Studies show that the benefit of taking statins in reducing heart attack death is no better than taking an aspirin a day, plus, there are no benefits of people taking statins past the age of 65.

For those who still feel they need to take statins, at least supplement with vitamin K2, magnesium, and ubiquinol to prevent heart failure and death.

High Blood Pressure

BLOOD PRESSURE IS the measure of systolic and diastolic pressures, and noted by saying something like my blood pressure was 120 over 80. These are the forces exerted by the heart on the arterial blood vessel walls. **Systolic pressure** is the maximum height that the fully contracted heart muscle would raise mercury (scientific symbol—Hg) in a glass column, in millimeters (mm).

Diastolic pressure is the residual level of mercury in that same glass column when the heart is relaxed; or the residual pressure on the artery wall, also measured in mm of Hg. This measuring system stems from the first method of testing blood pressure, where the height in mm of an actual glass column of mercury represented blood pressure.

Today, pneumatic and electronic devices have replaced the need for mercury columns, but the values still represent the equivalent of those first test methods as depicted by mm Hg.

The normal range for resting blood pressure is 120/80 mm Hg, but can vary greatly depending on activity. When performing physical activity, the blood pressure can be well over 120/80 mm Hg. Therefore, rest while sitting for five minutes before measuring blood pressure—even standing, the blood pressure will be higher. Have your blood pressure monitored regularly by trained healthcare providers since long-term hypertension (high blood pressure) is a risk factor for heart disease and strokes.

The American Heart Association (AMA) designates risk of hypertension with the blood pressure measurement, as follows:

Blood Pressure (mm Hg)	AMA Classification
120 to 139 over 80 to 90	pre-hypertension
140 to 179 over 90 to 110	hypertension
systolic pressure over 180	severe hypertension

Again, these are significant values when the person is at rest. A pressure reading of 155/104 mm Hg while playing a rigorous game of basketball, does not mean you are hypertensive—but if that is the pressure at rest, seek medical attention now!

Many other conditions associate with hypertension as part of metabolic syndrome; it is concomitant in 75 percent of stroke victims, 50 percent of heart attack victims, and 50 percent of diabetics. Thus, it is critical to maintain a healthy blood pressure to reduce the interrelated effects of metabolic syndrome. Hypertension also increases risk of kidney failure, eye problems, and visceral fat (beer gut).

As with most other diseases, excessive accumulation of free radicals and lipid peroxidation products is a central cause of hypertension via inflammation. Lipid peroxidation is the process through which free radicals take electrons from the lipids in our cell membranes, resulting in cell damage and more production of free radicals.

Hypertension results from two different consequences of inflammation. The first is when the free radical damage occurs in

CHAPTER SEVEN | A LOOK AT COMMON DISEASES

the brainstem on the parasympathetic nervous system that controls blood pressure. The cell damage to neural transmitter synapses will cause a rise in blood pressure from uncontrolled contraction of the smooth muscle cells in arterial walls. When the arterial walls constrict, this decreases the volume of blood that can pass through and correspondingly increases blood pressure.

The second way inflammation causes high blood pressure is that free radicals cause damage to the artery cell wall lining. This results in loss of arterial cell wall elasticity, causing rigidity, which increases blood pressure.

This concept is analogous to why plumbers place expansion tanks in closed-loop hot-water systems to prevent an excessive and damaging water pressure increase that would burst pipes. The expansion tank provides "elasticity" in the plumbing system to prevent damage.

Loss of vessel elasticity also increases risk for strokes, aneurysms, heart attacks, renal failure, loss of vision, and atherosclerosis.

To control high blood pressure, practice the same measures to reduce and prevent inflammation. Limit intake of refined sugar, HFCS, and high glycemic food consumption. Substitute omega-3 oils for omega-6 oils. Utilize supplements that provide antioxidants. Eat plenty of healthy vegetables and fruits. Reduce life's stress initiators, exercise, and get plenty of sleep. By this point, the basic preventive protocols should be like listening to a tape playing on a continuous loop!

Antihypertensive medications, such as Lisinopril®, Atenolol®, Tenormin®, and Hydrochlorothiazide®, that treat high blood pressure, have side effects. The side effects vary, but the common ones are depletion of magnesium and ubiquinol (CoQ10), plus the increased frustration in older men (and their spouses) from erectile dysfunction.

Arrhythmias

ARRHYTHMIAS ARE CONDITIONS in which the heartbeat is irregular in rhythm, too fast, or too slow. It may involve palpitations or the feeling of skipping a beat. Most types of arrhythmias are not serious, but some can result in cardiac arrest and death. Arrhythmias affect 2 to 3 percent of the population, and the affliction risk increases with age.

Two types of arrhythmias are atrial and ventricular fibrillation. Atrial fibrillation (A-fib) is rapid and irregular beating of the atria of the heart (heart flutter), which can lead to incomplete filling of the ventricles. The two heart atria fill the respective two ventricles, where one ventricle pumps blood to lungs while the other ventricle pumps blood to the rest of the body. A-fib usually is not fatal but it can be debilitating.

Ventricular fibrillation (V-fib) is the uncoordinated and incomplete contraction of the ventricles, which leads to partial perfusion of the lungs resulting in diminished blood oxygenation, as well as decreased blood flow to the rest of the body. If the brain receives too little and/or low-oxygenated blood, the brain will initiate fainting to get the head lower than the heart, to obtain more blood and oxygen.

V-fib is the most common and more serious in cardiac arrest victims and is why it is important to start CPR (cardiopulmonary resuscitation) and initiate the use of an AED (automated external

CHAPTER SEVEN | A LOOK AT COMMON DISEASES

defibrillator). The AED assesses the victim for irregular ventricular fibrillations, which may require a "shock" to reset the electrical conduction in the heart and obtain regular heartbeats. Without this electrical reset, the patient will die in a matter of minutes due to lack of oxygen to the brain.

Glutamate receptors found in the brain facilitate neurotransmission. Since neurotransmission is universal within the body, these receptors also occur in every organ—even the heart and blood vessels. The neural bundle that transmits the electrical impulse through the heart muscle contains glutamate receptors for normal nerve conduction. As with the brain, normal glutamate levels create proper nerve function, but excessive levels can over stimulate heart muscle fibers and lead to arrhythmias and death.

The elemental hero that once again prevents glutamate's zealous damage is magnesium. It prevents the heart's over-excitability, and thus arrhythmias, by blocking the glutamate receptors. Magnesium also helps reduce inflammation and raises glutathione levels in heart muscle thereby protecting the heart from free radical damage. The combination of high glutamate consumption and low magnesium levels in 75 percent of the population is potentially deadly. Antihypertensive and diuretic drugs that deplete magnesium can further promote arrhythmias.

To help prevent arrhythmias, it is imperative to eliminate MSG from the diet. This also means no aspartame from diet soda pop that converts into glutamate. In addition, sugar should be limited to that found naturally in fruits—that is, no added refined sugar.

Protocols for Heart Disease

HERE AGAIN, WE want to avoid foods that promote inflammation such as MSG, refined sugar, and omega-6 fats. Utilize inflammation-reducing supplements such as curcumin, quercetin, vitamin E, magnesium, ellagic acid (berries), DHA, and vitamin D3. Heart failure patients have common deficiencies in selenium, zinc, magnesium, B1 (thiamine), and B2 (riboflavin), which are alleviated by a healthy diet and supplementation. PQQ (pyrroloquinoline quinone) can reduce the heart damage to the affected ischemic heart muscle and therefore administer it as soon as possible after a heart attack. Avoiding statin drugs is also important for the reasons previously stated. Consult with your healthcare provider to coordinate these supplements with prescription heart drugs.

Supplement Protocols for Atherosclerosis

THE BEST WAY TO avoid atherosclerotic plaques is to prevent them from forming in the first place. However, if plaques have already formed in the blood vessels, maintenance in a stable state prevents blockage of the vessel.

The best approach promotes prevention and strengthening the fibrous cap over the atherosclerotic plaque so it will not rupture and create blood clots. The following supplements and their increase in dosage will help prevent and stabilize atherosclerotic plaques.

Liposomal C (vitamin C)—take 1000 mg (two capsules) every two hours until six grams are taken per day. It promotes collagen and vessel integrity, as well as strengthens the fibrous cap to prevent rupture and clotting. It reduces atherosclerosis and thus reduces heart attacks and strokes.

Magnesium—take 425 mg (three tablets) three times per day, and get your red blood cell (RBC) essential minerals test to maintain proper cellular levels. Low magnesium allows oxidized LDL cholesterol to enter the blood vessel endothelial cells and cause inflammation. Magnesium stops this inflammation by inhibiting the calcium-triggered inflammation pathways in the cells. Thus, proper magnesium levels prevent calcium build-up in the blood vessel walls and the resulting atherosclerotic plaques.

Aged Garlic Extract—take 600 mg (two capsules), one in the morning and another in the evening. It works within 3 hours and lasts 4 to 6 hours. As a powerful antioxidant, it reverses the build-up of atherosclerotic plaques, as noted by a UCLA Medical Center study. View the research study at http://www.newsmax.com/Health/Headline/garlic-heart-disease-plaque/2014/05/06/id/569839/.

Some claim that aged garlic extract works better than statins to combat atherosclerosis. Aged garlic also dissolves blood clots and thins blood, which is important for diabetics who have a high incidence of heart attacks and strokes due to clots forming from atherosclerotic plaques. It increases good HDL cholesterol and prevents the oxidation of bad LDL cholesterol. Garlic at this dosage is very safe; toxic levels are above 20,000 mg.

Borage Oil (GLA—gamma linolenic acid)—take 1300 mg (one softgel) twice per day. This anti-inflammatory agent prevents blood vessel inflammation that would produce the atherosclerotic plaque.

CLA (conjugated linoleic acid)—take 2400 mg (three softgels) twice per day. It lowers LDL (better than a statin drug, with no side effects) and more importantly, it lowers triglycerides that are the main causative agent for atherosclerosis. CLA reduces inflammation by reducing blood vessel cell wall damage and is protective from atherosclerosis by preventing LDL and omega-6 fats from oxidizing.

Curcumin—take 400 mg (one capsule) three times per day. This powerful antioxidant decreases the oxidation of LDL cholesterol and reverses atherosclerosis.

DHA (Docosahexaenoic acid)—take 560 mg (two softgels) three times daily with food. It decreases inflammation and the resulting atherosclerotic plaque.

Grape Seed Extract—take 100 mg (one capsule) twice daily. It helps stabilize atherosclerotic plaques in blood vessels so part of the plaque will not break off and create blockage (blood clot) downstream.

L-Carnosine—take 500 mg (one capsule) twice daily. As an antioxidant, carnosine helps prevent and dissolve AGE's, which reduces atherosclerosis.

PQQ (pyrroloquinoline quinone)—take 10 mg (one capsule) twice daily. PQQ can reduce the heart damage to heart muscle fibers from lack of blood flow (and thus low oxygen) so it should be given as soon as possible after a heart attack.

Quercetin with Bromelain—take 500 mg (two capsules) three times per day. This anti-inflammatory agent prevents and reduces atherosclerotic plaque build-up. As a powerful antioxidant, quercetin prevents the oxidation of LDL cholesterol. It also prevents heart attacks and strokes.

Taurine—take 500 mg (one capsule) twice daily. It acts as an anti-inflammatory agent that reduces LDL cholesterol from entering the blood vessel wall. If LDL cannot enter the vessel wall, it will not oxidize, and thus it prevents atherosclerosis from occurring in the first place. It also prevents AGE's and the resulting chronic inflammation. Taurine can reduce blood sugar levels so for those with reactive hypoglycemia, it should be taken along with a meal. Otherwise, take it 30 minutes before a meal.

Ubiquinol—take 100 mg (one softgel) twice daily. It is the active and more bio-available supplement form of CoQ10.

It is part of the antioxidant network that protects the cell membranes (lipid bilayers) against lipid peroxidation and damage, which prevents inflammation in the blood vessels and atherosclerotic plaques.

Supplement Protocols for High Blood Pressure

HIGH BLOOD PRESSURE can be reduced by proper diet, exercise, sleep, and the reduction of stress. We have seen how many prescription drugs have detrimental side effects so it behooves us to seek a more natural approach.

Here is a list of those vitamins, minerals, and supplements that help decrease blood pressure, without harmful side effects.

Liposomal C (Vitamin C)—take 1000 mg (two capsules) every two hours until six grams are taken per day. Vitamin C protects the heart and strengthens blood vessel wall integrity by making them more elastic through collagen formation, which lowers blood pressure.

Magnesium—take 425 mg (three tablets) three times per day. Magnesium helps reduce inflammation associated with high blood pressure and helps protect the heart. Low magnesium is rampant among the population and contributes to death from sudden cardiac failure. Carbonated drinks, anti-hypertensive drugs, statin drugs, and extreme exercise can further deplete magnesium levels.

Aged Garlic Extract—take 600 mg (two capsules), one in the morning and another in the evening. It lowers blood pressure by relaxing blood vessels making them more elastic. As an antioxidant, it helps reduce the cause of chronic inflammation and the immune response.

Acetyl-L-Carnitine—take 500 mg (one capsule) twice daily. It improves function of the cells lining the blood vessels (endothelial cells), and thus lower blood pressure to help prevent heart attacks and strokes.

Curcumin—take 400 mg (one capsule) three times per day. An anti-inflammatory, it prevents inflammation of blood vessel walls and inhibits their rigidity.

Hawthorn—take 500 mg (one capsule) twice daily. It is the best alternative to anti-hypertensive drugs, as it lowers blood pressure by dilating blood vessels while strengthening blood vessels and heart muscle for stronger contractions. As an antioxidant, hawthorn protects the walls of major blood vessels from inflammation of omega-6 fats oxidation.

Synergistic effectiveness can occur with simultaneous prescription anti-hypertensive drugs. Therefore, lower the dosage of these prescription drugs with the help of your healthcare provider, and thereby reduce their harmful side effects.

The maximum dosage for Hawthorn is 1800 mg/day; we are

well short of this level.

Quercetin with Bromelain—take 500 mg (two capsules) three times per day. This anti-coagulant thins blood and lowers blood pressure.

Taurine—take 500 mg (one capsule) twice daily. It protects the heart and its function by regulating calcium levels and lowering blood pressure.

Ubiquinol—take 100 mg (one softgel) twice daily. This protects against omega-6 oxidation and inflammatory damage.

Supplement Protocols for Arrhythmias

ARRHYTHMIAS CAN RANGE from being annoying to scary and even deadly. Supplements can help eliminate or reduce their occurrence, but always seek the care of a cardiologist to make sure other factors are not involved. Supplement maintenance protocols are important to follow for basic heart protection. Some supplements will need to have the dosage increased.

The following list includes supplements at increased levels to which I would personally take if I had high blood pressure:

Magnesium—take 425 mg (three tablets) three times per day. Get the RBC essential mineral test to determine your magnesium levels. Magnesium reduces intra-vascular blood clotting and guards the heart against attacks, failure, arrhythmias, and muscle degeneration, all by decreasing inflammatory cytokines in the heart muscle.

Magnesium competes with glutamate and blocks glutamate receptors in the heart that cause excitotoxicity that would otherwise cause arrhythmias. People have arrhythmias, and many healthcare providers never even check their magnesium levels. I have asked patients with arrhythmias (and those taking statins or high blood pressure drugs), if they take magnesium. Unfortunately, most say no and that they haven't had their magnesium levels tested. Do not let this happen to you.

Acetyl-L-Carnitine—take 500 mg (one capsule) twice daily. Acetyl-L-carnitine helps prevent arrhythmias.

DHA (Docosahexaenoic acid)—take 560 mg (two softgels) three times daily with food. It decreases inflammation and glutamate toxicity by reducing the over activity of heart glutamate receptors and allows magnesium to better modulate electrical conduction to prevent arrhythmias.

Hawthorn—take 500 mg (one capsule) twice daily. It relieves heart failure and palpitations.

L-Carnosine—take 500 mg (one capsule) twice daily. It protects the heart and decreases arrhythmias.

Taurine—take 500 mg (one capsule) twice daily. This anti-inflammatory agent protects the heart.

References

CDC.gov – Heart Disease Facts, American Heart Association – 2015 Heart Disease and Stroke Update, compiled by AHA, CDC, NIH and other governmental sources.

McGill HC, McMahan CA, Gidding SS (March 2008). "Preventing heart disease in the 21st century: implications of the Pathobiological Determinants of Atherosclerosis in Youth (PDAY) study". *Circulation* 117 (9): 1216–27. PMID 18316498.

Blaylock, R.L., Blaylock wellness report, Sept 2013-sites a study by Alan Collins in Circulation Research, 2009, 104: e42-e54.

Finn AV, Nakano M, Narula J, Kolodgie FD, Virmani R (July 2010). "Concept of vulnerable/unstable plaque". Arterioscler. Thromb. Vasc. Biol. 30 (7): 1282–92.doi:10.1161/ATVBAHA.108.179739. PMID 20554950.

http://circres.ahajournals.org/content/104/6/e42.abstract.

"Understanding blood pressure readings". American Heart Association. *11 January 2011. Retrieved 30 March 2011.*

http://www.ncbi.nlm.nih.gov/pmc/articles/PMC2735432/.

http://www.cvphysiology.com/Blood%20Pressure/BP008.htm.

"What Is Arrhythmia?". http://www.nhlbi.nih.gov. July 1, 2011.

Zoni-Berisso, M; Lercari, F; Carazza, T; Domenicucci, S (2014). "Epidemiology of atrial fibrillation: European perspective.". *Clinical epidemiology* 6: 213–20.doi:10.2147/CLEP.S47385. PMID 24966695.

Strokes

THE SUDDEN DEATH of brain cells due to lack of oxygen is called a stroke, and it is the second-highest cause of death in this country after coronary artery disease (as of 2013). Strokes are known as a cerebral vascular accident (CVA) because it involves the brain's blood vessels.

A stroke may be due to either a *blockage* of blood flow to part of the brain, called ischemic CVA, or the *rupture* and bleeding of an artery in the brain, called hemorrhagic CVA. Either way it results in the lack of oxygen to brain cells, which causes their death. Brain cells can only last four to five minutes without oxygen before the cells die. This is a critical factor to remember when an unconscious victim is not breathing and needs CPR.

Since the affected artery supplies blood to a specific region of the brain, the stroke will affect only that portion. Signs and symptoms of the stroke often develop quickly, but might take hours or days to appear and depend upon the area of the brain impaired. The severity and length of affliction vary among different people.

Indications may be a sudden weakness or paralysis of one side of the body. Parts of the face, arms, or legs could become numb. The victim could have trouble speaking, seeing, breathing, or walking. One could even experience a sudden severe headache and maybe the loss of consciousness.

The main risk factor for a stroke is *high blood pressure that causes the rupture or tear of the arterial wall, seen in hemorrhagic strokes*. The resulting brain bleed does not allow oxygen to get into the brain cells. Atherosclerosis will cause the *ischemic stroke where the plaque breaks away from the arterial wall and blocks the vessel downstream, causing diminished oxygenation of nerve cells*. Other risk factors are obesity, diabetes, atrial fibrillation, and smoking.

Death rates are about equal for ischemic and hemorrhagic strokes even though 87 percent of strokes are ischemic. Thus, the hemorrhagic stroke has a worse prognosis and is more deadly. If you have one stroke, you are likely to have a second within five years. As one would guess, aging is associated with increased risk; two thirds of all strokes occur in people over 65 years old. *The sad statistic is that half of the people who had a stroke live for less than one year because of the debilitating effects or recurrence of more strokes. This makes prevention extremely important and immediate treatment following a stroke critical.*

If you suspect you or someone else is having a stroke, call 9-1-1 immediately. Do not drive to the emergency room or hospital. Call an ambulance so that medical trained personnel can begin life-saving treatment. During a stroke, every minute counts.

Preventive and curative supplementation measures used for high blood pressure and atherosclerosis will assist dramatically to reduce risk for strokes. In fact, the Garden of Eden Lifestyle and diet, along with supplementation and exercise already mentioned, will provide the best way to prevent strokes. We will examine measures, in other sections, to prevent and curtail obesity and diabetes, which also have profound affects to reduce strokes.

Blood thinners such as gingko biloba and aged garlic extract can mitigate the ischemic stroke involving blood clots; they also help remove atherosclerotic plaques from blood vessels.

It is imperative to deliver immediate treatment within the first few hours. The faster the clots dissolve determines how severe the long lasting effects will be. Hemorrhagic strokes may require surgical intervention to lessen long-term effects. You will not know which type of stroke is present, so obtain immediate healthcare.

Since hemorrhagic strokes produce higher fatality rates, prevention is essential. French researchers report that people with a vitamin C deficiency have increased risk for hemorrhagic strokes. The reason is two-fold. First, vitamin C helps regulate and reduce blood pressure by dilating blood vessels. Reduced blood pressure exerts less force on blood vessels and decreases the chance of rupture. Second, vitamin C is required for the biosynthesis of collagen, which is the material that keeps blood vessels flexible and elastic. Thus, the vessels are more resistant to rupture because of a stronger cell matrix.

People with higher vitamin C levels reduced the risk of hemorrhagic stroke by 40 percent. In addition, people who ate vegetables six to seven days a week, had 54 percent less chance of a stroke than those who ate vegetables just two days or less per week.

Both ischemic and hemorrhagic strokes result from chronic inflammation. With the progression of inflammation, the severity of stroke can increase. Small strokes can lead to larger strokes due to worsening inflammation and the immune response of the surrounding brain tissue by the microglia.

The amount of chronic inflammation can be assessed by a blood test—using high-sensitivity C-reactive protein (hs-CRP). It does not tell you where the inflammation is located, only that you have it. Nevertheless, awareness is the first step to alleviate the problem.

Brain inflammation can be the result of excess iron, an excitotoxin that causes damage from free radicals. Excess iron has been shown to cause more devastating strokes—this may be why post-menopausal women have more deadly strokes than men, due to lack of menstruation ridding the body of iron. Alpha lipoic acid binds and removes toxic metals like iron and mercury, so it helps in the after effects of strokes by reducing excitotoxins in the brain.

Low magnesium levels are associated with inflammation and the increased damage from free radicals. Proper magnesium levels reduces inflammation, improve brain blood flow, increases antioxidant effectiveness, and blocks excitotoxicity.

CHAPTER SEVEN | A LOOK AT COMMON DISEASES

The good news is that strokes among American seniors are declining, but according to an article written in Newsmax Health (January 9, 2016), there is a "dramatic increase in strokes hitting the middle-agers." They report a 53 percent increase of stroke incidence in Americans aged 15 to 44. The number of stroke deaths is declining because the younger people are more likely to survive, but they are none-the-less affected and disabled. Factors that lead to more strokes in younger people are earlier onset of obesity, diabetes, and high blood pressure. According to Dr. Hoffman in the article, "Early attention to risk factors can dramatically minimize your risk" and 80 percent of strokes are preventable.

Supplement Protocols for Strokes

THE PREVENTIVE REGIMEN of supplements, diet, and exercise will greatly decrease the risk of stroke. If by chance you or a loved one develops a stroke, get immediate attention for optimal prognosis. It is better to go to the emergency room and find out you are fine, than to shrug it off and suffer debilitating effects or even death.

After initial treatment from medical personnel, increased supplementation of selective agents given soon thereafter will help alleviate the long lasting detrimental effects of strokes. The increased dosage of the following supplements should help those suffering a stroke.

Liposomal C (vitamin C)—take 1000 mg (two capsules) every two hours until six grams are taken per day. Vitamin C is very important as it decreases inflammation, is an antioxidant, and aids micro-vascular blood flow. It would be best to receive mega doses of IV vitamin C while in the hospital since it reduces the extent of stroke damage and initiates repair.

Magnesium—take 425 mg (three tablets) three times per day. Magnesium inhibits inflammation by blocking glutamate receptors, which inhibits excitotoxicity. It increases antioxidant effectiveness and improves blood flow in the brain.

Aged Garlic Extract—take 600 mg (two capsules), one in the morning and another in the evening. Aged garlic extract dissolves blood clots and thins blood, which is important for diabetics who have a high incidence of heart attacks and strokes due to clots forming from atherosclerotic plaques. It lowers blood pressure by relaxing blood vessels. It also protects the brain from inflammatory excitotoxins like mercury by binding and removing it from the body.

Acetyl-L-Carnitine—take 500 mg (one capsule) twice daily. It readily passes through the blood-brain barrier and protects brain cells by stimulating mitochondria to increase energy output. It also improves blood vessel cells to lower blood pressure and prevent strokes. Acetyl-L-carnitine is a powerful anti-inflammatory agent that if taken soon after a stroke, can protect brain cells and reduce damage by decreasing brain glutamate levels around the stroke site.

Curcumin—take 400 mg (one capsule) three times per day. This anti-inflammatory prevents inflammation of the brain after a stroke. It also stimulates wound healing and DNA repair, and increases mitochondrial energy.

DHA (Docosahexaenoic acid)—take 560 mg (two softgels) three times daily with food. It mitigates the effects of strokes on patients by decreasing brain inflammation and glutamate toxicity; take this as soon as possible after a stroke. It also improves brain blood flow to promote faster healing. Note that flaxseed, a beneficial adjunct, converts into DHA.

Grape Seed Extract—take 100 mg (one capsule) twice daily. It is a powerful antioxidant and anti-inflammatory that protects the brain from glutamate. It also decreases the absorption of iron, the free radical generator.

Hawthorn—take 500 mg (one capsule) two times per day. Hawthorn protects the brain against stroke damage by reducing brain inflammation. It reduces blood pressure by dilating blood vessels and strengthens blood vessels to prevent rupture.

Synergistic effectiveness can occur with simultaneous prescription anti-hypertensive drugs. Therefore, lower the dosage of these prescription drugs with the help of your healthcare provider, and thereby reduce their harmful side effects.

NAC (N-acetyl cysteine)—take 600 mg (one capsule) twice daily. It replenishes glutathione, the powerful antioxidant network heavy hitter. It performs its antioxidant role in the cell nucleus and cytoplasm mitochondria and protects from free radicals. Glutathione also chelates mercury, aluminum, and excess iron.

PQQ (pyrroloquinoline quinone)—take 10 mg (one capsule) twice daily. The most profound feature of PQQ is the maintenance and synthesis of more mitochondria. This is vital in situations where mitochondria become damaged by strokes.

Quercetin with Bromelain—take 500 mg (two capsules) three times per day. It is an anti-inflammatory agent that helps prevent strokes and lessens the after effect damage. Quercetin also chelates iron and increases mitochondrial energy, which stimulates healing, and repair of brain cells.

Taurine—take 500 mg (one capsule) twice daily. This anti-inflammatory agent protects the brain by decreasing excitotoxicity after stroke damage. Taurine can reduce blood sugar levels so for those with reactive hypoglycemia, it should be taken along with a meal. Otherwise, take it 30 minutes before a meal.

Ubiquinol—take 100 mg (one softgel) twice daily. It is the active and more bio-available supplement form of CoQ10. It protects against omega-6 fats oxidation and inflammatory damage of cell membranes and helps regenerate other antioxidants. Ubiquinol is also an essential component of the mitochondrial energy production process to stimulate cellular functions.

Vinpocetine—take 10 mg (one capsule) twice daily. A special property of vinpocetine increases blood flow in the brain's arterioles, even to areas damaged by strokes. This occurs without decreasing blood pressure. It also makes RBC's more flexible so they can navigate into small capillaries and oxygenate those areas to prevent cell death, especially after a stroke.

It also increases brain energy but does not increase free radical production, so it reduces inflammation and excitotoxicity. It even reduces the effect of released glutamate over activity from excitotoxicity, but allows normal glutamate receptors to function for neurotransmission.

Giving Vinpocetine directly after a stroke can protect stroke victims from brain damage, especially in the hippocampus (the memory/learning center).

References

http://www.nhlbi.nih.gov/health/health-topics/topics/stroke.

www.ncbi.nlm.nih.gov/pubmed/18468545.

"What Are the Signs and Symptoms of a Stroke?". http://www.nhlbi.nih.gov/health/health-topics/topics/stroke/signs.

"Who Is at Risk for a Stroke?". http://www.nhlbi.nih.gov/health/health-topics/topics/stroke/atrisk.

http://www.nydailynews.com/life-style/health/vitamin-linked-reduced-stroke-risk-article-1.1618380.

http://www.ncbi.nlm.nih.gov/pubmed/11022052.

www.researchgate.net/publication/11328158_Vinpocetine_increases_cerebral_blood_flow_and_oxygenation_in_stroke_patients_A_near_infrared_spectroscopy_and_transcranial_Doppler_study.

http://jonathanprouskynd.com/uploads/Myalgic_Encephalomyelitis_-_IHP.pdf.

Type 2 Diabetes

DIABETES IS THE Fifth leading cause of death in the U.S. In 2005, 23 million Americans had diabetes—and then it jumped to 26 million in 2015! That is almost a 9 percent increase in just 10 years. What is diabetes, and why is it so prevalent?

Diabetes is a disease whereby the body is unable to produce enough, or any, insulin, which causes the blood to have excess levels of sugar (**hyperglycemia**). This is detrimental to the body since the uptake of glucose from the blood, by cells—especially muscle cells—is critical for metabolism and survival.

There are three types of diabetes. **Type 1 diabetes** is also known as juvenile-onset diabetes or insulin-dependent diabetes. It is due to the inability of the body to produce any insulin and presents elevated blood sugar levels. **Type 3 diabetes** is a relatively new classification for diabetes that results in the brain from insulin resistance and is thought to promote Alzheimer's disease—we looked at this in the section pertaining to dementia. We will now look at the most common one, **Type 2 diabetes**, which accounts for close to 90 percent of all diabetes types.

Type 2 diabetes has steadily increased since the mid-twentieth century, along with obesity. In 1985, globally there were 30 million people diagnosed with Type 2 diabetes, and in 2010, it jumped to 285 million. It is common in the developed and developing countries, but is rare in the under-developed countries.

Could this be due to the ubiquity of refined sugar in the more developed countries, and the lack of its availability in the under-developed ones? I am sure the root cause in the United States is the standard American diet (how SAD it is), primarily due to the prevalence of sugar in our food products.

The World Health Organization (WHO) recognizes diabetes as a global epidemic.

Type 2 diabetes is also known as adult-onset diabetes, or non-insulin dependent diabetes. Hyperglycemia occurs here, too, but the cause is due to resistance of the tissue cells to respond to insulin, which inhibits sugar uptake within the cells, even though there is insulin present. The pancreas will secrete more insulin to counter balance the insulin resistance of tissue cells. With more insulin floating around, even the resistance of the cells should be overcome, right? Wrong. In fact, after long-term insulin resistance of tissue cells, the pancreas goes into hyper-drive to produce more insulin, but to no avail.

CHAPTER SEVEN | A LOOK AT COMMON DISEASES

With continued production leading to high insulin levels, more glucose and fatty acids are stored as fat, while fat itself is prevented from leaving the cells to be used as energy. When the insulin cannot bind to the cell wall to stimulate glucose uptake, the cell dies from lack of energy and the body will suffer fatigue. In time, because of over stimulation of insulin production and dysfunction of the pancreatic beta cells to produce insulin, levels will diminish and the person becomes insulin dependent, requiring insulin injections. The amount of insulin resistance versus beta cell dysfunction differs among individuals. Some people will have primarily insulin resistance and only a minor defect in insulin secretion, while others may have slight insulin resistance with a primary lack in insulin secretion.

So what causes the insulin resistance in the first place? A study by medical doctors Ralph DeFronzo and Devjit Tripathy published in the November 2009 issue of Diabetes Care, states that, "Insulin resistance in skeletal muscle is an early *metabolic defect* in the pathogenesis of Type 2 diabetes and that muscle lipid accumulation plays a central role in the etiology of the muscle insulin resistance." Because mitochondria oxidize fatty acids, any dysfunction to the mitochondria (metabolic defect) leads to an excess of intracellular fatty acids, which drives the increase in insulin resistance of the cell to diminish further sugar absorption. It is like trying to blow a balloon up with more air after it is fully inflated. The balloon (like the muscle cell) resists more air (sugar uptake due to increased insulin resistance). Thus, the thought is that mitochondrial dysfunction is the cause of muscle insulin resistance and Type 2 diabetes; it is also the cause of cancer as noted by the Warburg Effect. Wow, how interesting is that?

Another theory states, "It is unclear which is the cart and

which is the horse: mitochondrial dysfunction leading to increased muscle cell lipid content and insulin resistance, or increased muscle lipid content (i.e., secondary to elevated plasma free fatty acid levels and/or excessive lipid ingestion) leading to mitochondrial dysfunction and insulin resistance." It would seem that whichever way you look at it, inflammation and mitochondrial dysfunction are the root causes. We examined the influence of both on diseases in the section on aging. Inflammation will cause mitochondria dysfunction from free fatty acid oxidation; and consumption of unhealthy omega-6 fats will drive the mitochondrial dysfunction process to create inflammation. Also remember, the combination of sugar, fatty acids, and proteins create AGE's.

Symptoms of Type 2 diabetes are increased thirst, which leads to more frequent urination, and increased hunger (not surprising if sugar is not absorbed by cells for fuel—the body induces eating until it is nourished). It is often associated with itchiness, vision problems, bruising, fatigue, and peripheral neuropathy (dysfunction of extremity nerves causing numbness, weakness, or pain). Long-term complications can lead to shortened life span, heart disease, strokes, atherosclerosis, blindness, kidney failure, frequent infections, impotence, poor circulation in limbs requiring amputation, and cancer.

The cause of diabetes Type 2 can be linked to lifestyle and genetics, both of which lead to inflammation and mitochondrial dysfunction. Lifestyle factors that stimulate this condition are inactivity leading to excessive weight, poor diet, stress, lack of sleep that affects metabolism, and even smoking. Sugar is the main dietary component, along with omega-6 fats, that increases the risk. To diminish these effects we can change our lifestyle factors.

CHAPTER SEVEN | A LOOK AT COMMON DISEASES

Eating a healthy diet that reduces refined sugar and high glycemic foods, as well as avoiding omega-6 fats will diminish the effects of diabetes. Exercise consisting of both HIIT and HIST will increase insulin sensitivity and promote healthy mitochondria to alleviate diabetic affects.

More than 36 genes influence the increased risk of becoming a Type 2 diabetic. Some of the genetic variations probably involve impairing the function of mitochondria. Even though the genetic factors can't be reversed, their effects can be mitigated through lifestyle changes.

Diabetics have high levels of inflammation due to glucose-induced free radicals and lipid peroxidation products. There are also high levels of AGE's in the red blood cells to impair cell function and enzymes. These cause the diabetic's secondary afflictions of obesity and high blood pressure. Because these conditions are interrelated and due to a metabolism disorder, they are grouped together as "metabolic syndrome," which also includes high blood levels of free fatty acids, as seen in diabetics. *The presence of any one of the conditions leads to a greater risk of having the other(s), as the underlying cause is the same.*

Sugar, especially HFCS, greatly enhances inflammation by promoting insulin resistance, which keeps blood sugar levels high. This promotes free radical production and inflammation leading to atherosclerosis, cardiovascular disease, and increased risk for hypertension, obesity, and even cancer. An important fact to remember is that diabetic patients will develop atherosclerosis even when cholesterol levels are normal or even low. The oxidation of the excessive omega-6 fats in the blood leads to vascular inflammation and plaque build-up.

So what happens when we consume sugar? The first thing that happens is that sugar makes us crave more food and sugar. Sugar is even more addicting than cocaine. Refined sugar triggers the brain's natural opioid release, and we feel great from that "sugar high." Food manufacturers know this and add sugar whenever possible. No wonder the rates of diabetes are increasing and at earlier ages in children.

The American Heart Association recommends limiting your daily added sugar intake to nine teaspoons (38 grams) for men and six teaspoons (25 grams) for women. However, this is still too much and can promote cancer. It is better for both men and women to limit the amount of total sugar intake to 25 grams or less per day from all sources, not just added sugar. Most fruits have sugar in the form of fructose in them—but it is still sugar. Limit total sugar from fruits to that in about one cup per day.

Other concerns for sugar consumption include loss of cognitive flexibility and impairment of both long and short-term memory. Sugar is an excitotoxin that causes brain inflammation and affects brain function.

To counteract the effects of diabetes, we have looked at the hormone, insulin, which stimulates the uptake of glucose into tissue cells. Insulin regulation is critical to maintain blood glucose levels in a steady state, to induce the burning of sugar as fuel and deter its storage as fat. This was the first secret to develop a leaner, stronger body while avoiding cancer and other diseases.

Let's also review two other hormones, leptin and adiponectin. Leptin induces glucose absorption into cells via insulin stimulation, and adiponectin increases fat utilization for oxidation and decreases insulin resistance, which drives more glucose into cells. Thus, both are synergistic and increase metabolism. Mice studies have also shown these two hormones to reverse insulin resistance.

Adiponectin levels in humans show reduced levels in diabetics compared to non-diabetics—thus, more fat is stored leading to obesity because of increased insulin resistance. Increasing adiponectin levels can help those with Type 2 diabetes to curb their appetite, which will also decrease the chance of obesity. In the next section, we will look more closely at how adiponectin counteracts obesity.

Protocols for Diabetes

PHYSICIANS HAVE USED prescription drugs to treat diabetes over the years. Our goal here is to use a healthy diet and exercise to decrease or eliminate dependency on drugs, which also avoids their hazardous side effects. Exercise can be anything from walking, swimming, sport activities, to HIIT and HIST, as we discussed in Chapter Six—The Garden of Eden Lifestyle; A Practical Paradigm Shift.

A healthy diet would include the suggestions previously made and would start with the maintenance levels for supplementation. Also, eat your vegetables, which provide necessary dietary fiber. Keep in mind they have over 5,000 phytonutrients that are powerful antioxidants important in reducing inflammation and preventing LDL oxidation. They even improve immunity, aid detoxification, and—best of all for diabetics—they help lower blood sugar.

As in our earlier discussion of cancer, *reduction of both*

refined and natural sugar is critical. If you must eat sugar, stay with natural sugar and consume it later in the meal; this helps dilute the sugar and lowers its glycemic effect.

For more benefit in making dietary changes to correct diabetes, lean toward a ketogenic diet with MCT oil, flaxseed oil, and the use of omega-3 oils (coconut oil, olive oil, palm kernel oil). Get a blood test for the essential fatty acid profile, which will assess the amount of omega-6 and omega-3 oils present in the blood. The desired ratio of omega-6 fats to omega-3 fats is five-to-one or less, the smaller the ratio the better. The omega-6 oils you should drastically reduce are safflower, sunflower, canola, corn, and peanut; eliminate soy totally.

You may initially experience episodes of diminished energy, irritability, and sugar craving while eating a reduced carbohydrate diet. Hang in there! Those symptoms will go away within a week or two, leaving you with more energy than before. The sugar cravings will disappear too, and this will greatly suppress the problems associated with diabetes. Fresh vegetables and fruits will even taste better and further promote your good health. It will take time to transition, so just be patient.

Studies show diabetics have an excess of iron, which, if not bound to red blood cells can be a source of free radical production and inflammation. Diabetics should reduce iron consumption by eating less red meat and avoiding vitamin C with meals that binds and absorbs more iron into the body.

Ellagic acid from eating berries will also help decrease visceral inflammation from iron's free radicals.

Some supplements in the maintenance protocol are very beneficial to alleviate diabetic effects. EGCG from green tea extract reduces visceral inflammation, and vitamin E helps protect from AGE's. Pycnogenol protects fragile blood vessels that could otherwise lead to strokes and gangrene.

Supplement Protocols for Type 2 Diabetes

DIABETES IS ONE condition of metabolic syndrome that influences and promotes the others (high blood pressure, obesity, and elevated blood levels of free fatty acids) as well as the non-metabolic syndrome disease we know as cancer. Therefore, it is imperative to maintain control over diabetes and its deleterious effects. The following supplements with their higher doses, above the standard maintenance levels, are the ones I would take to reduce the effects of diabetes. Work with your healthcare provider to minimize or eliminate the need for prescription drugs.

Liposomal C (vitamin C)—take 1000 mg (two capsules) every two hours until six grams are taken per day. Vitamin C is very important as it decreases inflammation, is an antioxidant, and aids in the prevention of other metabolic syndrome conditions. Do not take it with meals or iron to prevent excessive absorption of iron. It can also interfere with vitamin B12 uptake, so stagger ingestion of both.

Vitamin D3—take 10,000 IU (two softgels) twice daily. It improves insulin levels, lowers blood sugar, and improves insulin resistance. Thus, it reduces the chance of developing Type 2 diabetes and the resulting inflammation. Studies have shown that low levels of vitamin D3 are associated with increased risk of developing diabetes.

Have your blood level tested; the desired target is around 90 ng/ml. Have the test performed in the winter and during the summer. Exposure to sunlight in the summer can boost vitamin D3 levels so that less supplementation is required. Conversely, winter months would necessitate greater supplementation.

Magnesium—take 425 mg (three tablets) three times per day. Magnesium helps reduce inflammation by reversing insulin resistance. With more glucose absorbed into muscle tissue, an insulin steady state occurs. Magnesium decreases risk for peripheral neuropathy and metabolic syndrome in general.

Aged Garlic Extract—take 600 mg (two capsules), one in the morning and another in the evening. It is an antioxidant that helps reduce the cause of chronic inflammation and the immune response from excessive blood sugar levels and AGE's.

Alpha lipoic acid—take 250 mg twice daily. This powerful antioxidant stimulates cells to produce energy via mitochondria while lowering blood sugar by improving insulin efficiency, thus increasing muscle cell uptake of glucose. The dramatic effect is to overcome the mitochondrial dysfunction by protecting and repairing mitochondria from aging, the suspected cause of Type 2 diabetes. Alpha lipoic acid also decreases peripheral neuropathy, the debilitating painful tingling in the body's extremities.

Supplementation with alpha lipoic acid may take up to three months to obtain results. As noted before, due to the ability of alpha lipoic acid to increase glucose uptake in the cells, I encourage caution to those susceptible to reactive hypoglycemia. This is the condition where excessive insulin release during a high glycemic meal causes a rebound low blood sugar level (hypoglycemia), which can be dangerous and even fatal. Seek professional healthcare to monitor proper blood glucose levels.

Alpha lipoic acid will also deplete biotin levels; therefore maintain adequate supplementation of biotin as well.

CLA (conjugated linoleic acid)—take 2400 mg (three softgels) twice daily. It reduces inflammation and helps reduce visceral fat with associated inflammatory cytokines. CLA aids in preventing other conditions of metabolic syndrome as well.

Curcumin—take 400 mg (one capsule) three times per day. This anti-inflammatory prevents inflammation and increases mitochondrial energy. Curcumin reduces visceral inflammation and reduces AGE's.

DHA (Docosahexaenoic acid)—take 560 mg (two softgels) three times daily with food. It decreases inflammation. Flaxseed, a beneficial adjunct, converts into DHA.

PQQ (pyrroloquinoline quinone)—take 10 mg (one capsule) twice daily. The most profound feature of PQQ is the maintenance and synthesis of more mitochondria, which can be vital in situations where mitochondrial damage is due to inflammation. Healthy mitochondria prevent insulin resistance and mitigate the effects of diabetes.

Quercetin with Bromelain—take 500 mg (two capsules) three times per day. This anti-inflammatory agent increases mitochondrial energy and reduces visceral inflammation, along with AGE's.

References

https://en.wikipedia.org/wiki/Diabetes_mellitus.

http://www.ncbi.nlm.nih.gov/pmc/articles/PMC3876339/.

http://thelancet.com/journals/landia/article/PIIS2213-8587(15)00316-2/fulltext.

http://www.ncbi.nlm.nih.gov/pmc/articles/PMC2811436/.

http://oregonstate.edu/ua/ncs/archives/2015/jun/fat-sugar-cause-bacterial-changes-may-relate-loss-cognitive-function.

http://www.ncbi.nlm.nih.gov/pubmed/22473784.

Obesity

OBESITY IS A condition characterized by the excessive accumulation and storage of fat in the body. It can have a negative impact on health and results in metabolic syndrome, cancer, and dementia. Research shows around one in five deaths in the United States are associated with obesity, accounting for 75 percent of healthcare costs. A global study in 2014 reported that obesity is responsible for an estimated 500,000 worldwide cancer cases each year.

Obesity is more common in adult women, but the rates for both men and women are soaring. Children have also seen a stark increase in obesity rates, and alarmingly, even those under five years of age are becoming more obese.

In the United States, a drastic increase in obesity transformed from 2.5 percent (6 million adults) in 2008 to a new high of 28 percent of the adult population in 2015. This is a fast growing health concern that promotes other ailments, declining work productivity, and lost wages from time off work. As reported by Scott Kahan, the director of the National Center for Weight & Wellness at George Washington University, the yearly cost of obesity is over $300 billion.

CHAPTER SEVEN | A LOOK AT COMMON DISEASES

In addition to the 28 percent of Americans who are obese, 35 percent of Americans are overweight, while just 35 percent have a normal weight. Studies have shown the increase in weight occurs most in those over age 65. The cause is aging and reduced thyroid function, which decreases metabolism and promotes obesity. Low thyroid production is also the leading cause of higher blood cholesterol levels and the reason why statins are not effective after age 65 to curb this trend.

African Americans are afflicted by obesity more than white or Asian Americans, but the sharpest increase in the rate is among white adults since 2008. The main culprit is overeating—taking in excessive calories from sugar-laden processed foods, unhealthy fats, and salt; a combination that encourages even more consumption . . . I'm hungry; pass the salted potato chips and soda pop, please. Oh, wait, never mind!

Obesity is the direct result of eating excessive amounts of carbohydrates. The term carbohydrate means any food that is particularly rich in the complex carbohydrate starch (such as cereal, bread and pasta) or simple carbohydrates, such as sugar (found in candy, jams, and desserts). The excessive amount of sugar eaten is then stored as glycogen and fat.

The leptin hormone regulates satiation, and the ghrelin hormone regulates hunger. However, insulin is the most important hormone for regulation of fat storage. Insulin regulates enzymes that store glucose and fatty acids in the fat cells, as well as the conversion of glucose into fatty acids that transform into triglycerides. High insulin levels drive more glucose and fatty acids into storage in the subcutaneous and visceral abdominal fat areas. Hence, the "spare tire" around the waist!

High consumption of carbohydrates (simple and complex) induces high insulin levels, and the higher the glycemic index and glycemic load, the higher the insulin level. Glycemic index *is the rate at which carbohydrates get absorbed into the blood, inducing a rise in insulin blood levels.* Low glycemic foods create a slow increase in blood sugar and corresponding lower insulin levels.

The goal for food consumption is to keep the blood sugar at low steady levels that do not create severe peaks and valleys of insulin that induce imbalances—the first secret to maintaining a lean and healthy body. This becomes even more pronounced when coupled with the third secret to a lean and healthy body—intermittent fasting–which decreases total calorie consumption and helps keep insulin at low steady state levels while reprograming the body to burn up fat stores.

Some people do not get fat no matter how much they eat because their muscle cell insulin receptors are very sensitive, while their fat cell receptors are resistant to insulin. They do not store glucose as fat but burn it in muscles, or store it as glycogen. This is why two different people who eat the same diet will react differently to fat storage. That's just not fair for most of us who, in just looking at food, gain weight! However, knowing the physiology behind the process allows us to overcome this obstacle.

Obesity can be quantified by using the popular method called body mass index (BMI). By definition, that is a person's weight divided by the square of their height. The following table shows values for different weight classifications.

BMI	Weight Classification
Greater than 39	Extremely obese
30 to 39	Obese
25 to 29	Overweight
18 to 24	Healthy weight
Less than 18	Underweight

BMI tables are the outcome of studies from population height and weight data. Please see the chart for your BMI values in Appendix C.

Keep in mind that BMI can be misleading, therefore use it as a guide only. For muscular men and women, the BMI value may report an overweight or obese issue, even though that person may be very fit and muscular to all appearances. A better method is to calculate percentage of body fat, which is a better indicator of risk for disease. This can be done using calipers or weight scales programmed to perform this function. Once the percent of body fat is calculated, compare it to values from the tables in Appendix B. There are two tables, one for women and one for men.

My personal values for BMI and percent body fat are 25 and 22, respectively. The value for BMI would indicate that I am slightly overweight; however, the body percent value has me placed in the middle of the ideal range. Thus, percent body fat is more accurate and measures actual body fat stored, while BMI does not take into account heavier individuals due to more muscle mass. *It generally boils down to how you look and feel, and we usually do not need calculations to tell us this.*

The cause of obesity is primarily linked to excessive poor diet intake with a lack of physical activity, while some cases are due to genetics, brain damage to the hypothalamus (the hunger regulatory center), and even psychological issues. In this section, we will discuss food intake, physical activity, and damage to the hypothalamus. The reader is encouraged to seek professional care for cases involving genetics and emotional stress issues.

The hypothalamus, which modulates hunger, lies just under the thalamus and above the brainstem. It links the nervous system to the endocrine system via the pituitary gland by secreting neurohormones to the pituitary gland. The hypothalamic hormones stimulate or inhibit secretion of pituitary hormones that regulate various body functions such as hunger.

If damage to the hypothalamus occurs during fetal development or later in life, the impact will disrupt the normal neurohormone flow and adversely affect hunger sensations leading to obesity. We have seen how MSG and artificial sweeteners can damage the hypothalamus. Once affected, the leptin satiation-hormone secretion level remains diminished, and overeating ensues from the abundance of the unregulated ghrelin hunger-hormone. Continued MSG in the diet compounds the problem further. It is imperative to read food labels and not consume these harmful food additives. Babies are four times more sensitive to MSG than are adults, another reason why the obesity rate for children under five is soaring.

Excessive intake of harmful foods will lead to obesity. In today's world, unfortunately we are inundated by junk food, GMO's, trans fats, processed foods, refined grains, MSG, and sugar. Unnecessary amounts of sugar have devastating effects. We have seen how blood sugar levels affect insulin levels in diabetics. Sugar also affects leptin resistance, leaving the body hungrier and inhibiting the burning of fat. The result is more hunger craving for

CHAPTER SEVEN | A LOOK AT COMMON DISEASES

the ever-addictive "sweet treats," which gets stored as visceral fat that, as we know, releases inflammatory cytokines. These cell-signaling proteins then generate chronic inflammation, metabolic syndrome, and even cancer. As if that isn't bad enough, the increased fat deposits turn off the adiponectin hormone, which further inhibits the metabolizing of fat as an energy source. This is a vicious downward obesity spiral—all from the effects of sugar.

Up to this point, we have used the word *sugar* to define any sweet-tasting carbohydrate. Technically speaking, glucose is the simple sugar metabolized in cells for energy. If it is not taken into cells, it will be stored as fat. Although this is already a bad scenario where excess glucose is stored as fat and causes obesity, fructose can be worse.

Refined table sugar, or sucrose, is comprised of two simple bound sugars—fructose and glucose. They are metabolically separated within our body. Glucose as we have seen increases the risk for diabetes. Fructose, however, is the more devastating component of table sugar and is also contained in fruits and especially in soda pop as HFCS. This is another reason to eliminate soda drinks from one's diet. Fructose absorption increases more dramatically when glucose is present than when it is alone.

The problem with fructose metabolism is the rapid creation of uric acid after consumption. Uric acid is a metabolic waste product found in the blood, and if not eliminated properly, it may cause gout. This debilitating disease results from uric acid crystals forming in joints, tendons, and surrounding tissues, causing intense pain. High uric acid levels inside cells act as pro-oxidants and damage the mitochondria. With malfunctioning mitochondria, insulin resistance increases, and little glucose is absorbed into cells for metabolism. The glucose is instead stored in fat cells without metabolizing chemical ATP. This is the reason obese people have little energy, but are at an increased risk for high blood pressure, diabetes, and kidney disease.

As a side note, have you wondered why over indulging in beer can cause the "beer belly" to appear? It turns out the yeast and other ingredients in beer work together to create more uric acid. This in turn leads to that spare tire around the middle from increased fat deposits.

Fructose can be a major component in various fruit juices, so read the product label carefully. Honey is also high in fructose and can be equivalent to HFCS.

So how much fructose can we safely consume? Today, 25 percent of all Americans consume over 134 grams of fructose daily. This consumption rate coincides with the statistic that 25 percent of Americans are either pre-diabetic or have Type 2 diabetes. It's not hard to see that we need to decrease fructose ingestion.

Nutrition counselors recommend that we keep total fructose below 25 grams per day. For those with cancer or any metabolic syndrome disorder, it is better to stay below 15 grams per day. As a reference, just one non-diet soda drink (12 ounces) would almost exceed your recommended daily limit.

Since fruits contain fructose, it is important to know which fruits have less fructose. See Appendix D for some common fruits and their fructose content. From this table, it is apparent that most fruits are relatively low in fructose. When you choose your favorite fruits, keep in mind the portion size and total fructose level so that you can stay below the recommended amount per day. Note that dried fruits have more concentrated fructose amounts so eating these can quickly put you over the limit.

The good news about eating fruits is the health benefit derived from the antioxidants and flavonoids, which help deter the harmful effects of fructose and glucose. Their fiber is also beneficial to help prevent colon cancer.

Protocols to Prevent Obesity

A PROPER DIET is crucial to reduce/prevent obesity. Sugar, both glucose and fructose, needs to be drastically reduced from the unhealthy average amount consumed today. The worst carbohydrates are from soda/fruit drinks, pasta, potato, pastry, bread, and ice cream. Review the internet for a list of lower glycemic foods to replace higher glycemic ones. Replace omega-6 fats with omega-3 fats, and use MCT oil to provide a source of metabolic energy that replaces sugar.

The blended vegetables/fruits mix shared with you above provides over 5,000 phytonutrients while providing fiber and very little carbohydrate. Consumption of the mix twice a day would go a long way to provide nutrients, slow sugar absorption, lower insulin levels, suppress hunger, and reduce total calories. A good alternative to baking with sugar is to use the all-natural plant-based Stevia. It is a natural sweetener.

Remember to eat organic whole foods that do not contain GMO's. Avoid processed meat like hot-dogs and cold cuts. As always, read food labels to avoid and eliminate MSG from your diet to prevent its toxic effects. The supplement taurine, along with magnesium, helps prevent the excitotoxic effects of MSG.

Increasing adiponectin hormone levels can help burn fat stores and reduce obesity. In the discussion of Type 2 diabetes, we learned how adiponectin also increases insulin sensitivity so more glucose consumption occurs in muscle cells and less converts into fat. It also facilitates the breakdown of fatty acids.

There are particular foods that increase adiponectin. Avocados are rich in monounsaturated fats that increase this hormone and are very tasty in salads. Olive oil, a healthy monounsaturated omega-3 fat, has polyphenols that cause the body to secrete adiponectin; it too, is a great addition to salads and replaces unhealthy omega-6 fats in salad dressings. Pumpkins and its seeds promote adiponectin. Another food that may surprise you for its health benefits is chocolate. However, I don't mean just any chocolate. It has to be dark chocolate with a high cocoa percentage. The higher the percentage the better as it has more flavonoids that stimulate adiponectin production. Be sure to look for cocoa percentages of 70 or more.

Exercise is extremely beneficial as well to combat obesity. From the section on exercise, we learned how myokines produced by muscle cells are anti-inflammatory and counter the effects of cytokines. Myokines benefit us in that they increase insulin sensitivity to promote glucose utilization in muscles. They also promote adiponectin in fat cells to liberate fat deposits for burning as fuel in muscles. HIIT and HIST are both beneficial in this regard.

Supplement Protocols for Obesity

OBESITY IS PART of the metabolic syndrome, and therefore any supplements that benefit high blood pressure and Type 2 diabetes

CHAPTER SEVEN | A LOOK AT COMMON DISEASES

will assist in reducing obesity. We will look at some additional supplements to ward off obesity.

Magnesium—take 425 mg (three tablets) three times per day. Get the RBC essential mineral test to determine your magnesium levels. Magnesium blocks glutamate receptors in the brain that would otherwise affect the hypothalamus and induce overeating.

CLA (conjugated linoleic acid)—take 800 mg (three softgels) twice daily, about one hour before a meal. It helps reduce harmful visceral fat and subcutaneous fat while gaining muscle mass.

Curcumin—take 400 mg (one capsule) three times per day. This anti-inflammatory reduces visceral inflammation and increases mitochondrial energy. Thus, it counteracts the buildup of uric acid in cells from fructose metabolism that damages the mitochondria. Curcumin lessens insulin resistance promoting the uptake of glucose into muscle while inhibiting its storage as fat.

DHA (Docosahexaenoic acid)—take 560 mg (two softgels) three times daily with food. It promotes adiponectin production and thereby reduces fat cells by inducing fatty acid breakdown while preventing fat production and storage.

PQQ (pyrroloquinoline quinone)—take 10 mg (one capsule) twice daily. It promotes the maintenance and synthesis of more mitochondria, which can be vital in situations where mitochondria are damaged due to uric acid buildup in cells. Healthy mitochondria prevent insulin resistance and the storing of glucose as fat.

Quercetin with Bromelain—take 500 mg (two capsules) three times per day. This anti-inflammatory agent increases mitochondrial energy and reduces visceral inflammation. Quercetin also lessens insulin resistance, promoting the uptake of glucose into muscle while inhibiting its storage as fat.

Conclusion

BY REDUCING SUGAR consumption, supplementing with important nutrients, fasting intermittently, and employing essential exercising we have effectively allowed our body to utilize the four secrets to obtain and maintain a healthy, lean body. This allows for low steady state blood sugar and insulin levels that hinder the fat storage of glucose while inhibiting overeating through supplementing with essential nutrients in sufficient quantities. The body also converts into a fat-burning machine through adhering to limited eating timeframes while assisted by effective exercising. All this happens without intense hunger—actually, with less hunger than before. Thus, I would hardly call this a "diet" at all! True insanity is doing the same thing repeatedly while expecting different results—and as such, diets become an exercise in insanity. What we really need is a paradigm shift and a new lifestyle—or truly returning to an earlier lifestyle that mimics the life and times of ancient people in the Garden of Eden. I have faith that YOU CAN DO THIS!

References

http://www.who.int/mediacentre/factsheets/fs311/en/.

Pianin, Eric. February, 18, 2016. "U.S. Obesity Rate Hit a Record High in 2015", The Fiscal Times.

http://ajph.aphapublications.org/doi/abs/10.2105/AJPH.2013.301379.

https://www.lewrockwell.com/2016/01/joseph-mercola/cancer-surge/.

http://articles.mercola.com/sites/articles/archive/2010/03/13/richard-johnson-interview.aspx.

Blaylock, R.L., Blaylock wellness report, Feb 2012.

EPILOGUE

I chose dentistry as a profession,
but I study nutrition out of necessity.

AS WE HAVE seen, the overall theme in this book is that inflammation is the cause of most diseases, and mitochondrial dysfunction is either the result of that inflammatory response or the cause itself. Without the mitochondrial powerhouse, the supply of chemical energy to cells fails, and tissues and organs become diseased. Therefore, it is crucial to bolster the immune system to combat inflammation and strengthen the mitochondria to prevent cellular disease. The methods to accomplish these tasks have been discussed in great detail.

The information in this book will remain relevant for all time. For all intents and purposes, human physiology will not change to render these principles meaningless any time soon. The only thing that will change will be more studies that prove the basis for a healthy body: good nutrition, proper supplementation, adequate exercise, and good sleep.

This is the key:

Eat a healthy diet, exercise, take life sustaining and healing supplements, sleep well, love, and dance—all the means of having and maintaining a healthy body and a happy life.

The proverbial fountain of youth is literally and figuratively in your hands—this book. What you decide to do with this information is up to you. Please choose wisely about your health—your life and well-being depend on it!

Peace be with you, and may God bless you.

APPENDIX A

Vaccine adjuvants as listed by the CDC website.

Adenovirus	sucrose, D-mannose, D-fructose, dextrose, potassium phosphate, plasdone C, anhydrous lactose, micro crystalline cellulose, polacrilin potassium, magnesium stearate, cellulose acetate phthalate, alcohol, acetone, castor oil, FD&C Yellow #6 aluminum lake dye, human serum albumin, fetal bovine serum, sodium bicarbonate, human-diploid fibroblast cell cultures (WI-38), Dulbecco's Modified Eagle's Medium, mono-sodium glutamate	March 2011
Anthrax (Biothrax)	aluminum hydroxide, benzethonium chloride, formaldehyde, amino acids, vitamins, inorganic salts and sugars	May 2012
BCG (Tice)	glycerin, asparagine, citric acid, potassium phosphate, magnesium sulfate, Iron ammonium citrate, lactose	February 2009
DT (Sanofi)	aluminum potassium sulfate, peptone, bovine extract, formaldehyde, thimerosal (trace), modified Mueller and Miller medium, ammonium sulfate	December 2005
DTaP (Daptacel)	aluminum phosphate, formaldehyde, glutaraldehyde, 2-Phenoxyethanol, Stainer-Scholte medium, modified Mueller's growth medium, modified Mueller-Miller casamino acid medium (without beef heart infusion), dimethyl 1-beta-cyclodextrin, ammonium sulfate	October 2013
DTaP (Infanrix)	formaldehyde, glutaraldehyde, aluminum hydroxide, polysorbate 80, Fenton medium (containing bovine extract), modified Latham medium (derived from bovine casein), modified Stainer-Scholte liquid medium	November 2013
DTaP-IPV (Kinrix)	formaldehyde, glutaraldehyde, aluminum hydroxide, Vero (monkey kidney) cells, calf serum, lactalbumin hydrolysate, polysorbate 80, neomycin sulfate, polymyxin B, Fenton medium (containing bovine extract), modified Latham medium (derived from bovine casein), modified Stainer-Scholte liquid medium	November 2013
DTaP-HepB-IPV (Pediarix)	formaldehyde, glutaraldehyde, aluminum hydroxide, aluminum phosphate, lactalbumin hydrolysate, polysorbate 80, neomycin sulfate, polymyxin B, yeast protein, calf serum, Fenton medium (containing bovine extract), modified Latham medium (derived from bovine casein), modified Stainer-Scholte liquid medium, Vero (monkey kidney) cells	November 2013
DTaP-IPV/Hib (Pentacel)	aluminum phosphate, polysorbate 80, formaldehyde, sucrose, gutaraldehyde, bovine serum albumin, 2-phenoxethanol, neomycin, polymyxin B sulfate, Mueller's Growth Medium, Mueller-Miller casamino acid medium (without beef heart infusion), Stainer-Scholte medium (modified by the addition of casamino acids and dimethyl-betacyclodextrin), MRC-5 (human diploid) cells, CMRL 1969 medium (supplemented with calf serum), ammonium sulfate, and medium 199	October 2013
Hib (ActHIB)	ammonium sulfate, formalin, sucrose, Modified Mueller and Miller medium	January 2014
Hib (Hiberix)	formaldehyde, lactose, semi-synthetic medium	March 2012
Hib (Pedvax-HIB)	aluminum hydroxphosphate sulfate, ethanol, enzymes, phenol, detergent, complex fermentation medium	December 2010

APPENDIX A (Continued)

Vaccine	Ingredients	Date
Hib/Hep B (Comvax)	yeast (vaccine contains no detectable yeast DNA), nicotinamide adenine dinucleotide, hemin chloride, soy peptone, dextrose, mineral salts, amino acids, formaldehyde, potassium aluminum sulfate, amorphous aluminum hydroxyphosphate sulfate, sodium borate, phenol, ethanol, enzymes, detergent	December 2010
Hib/Mening. CY (MenHibrix)	tris (trometamol)-HCl, sucrose, formaldehyde, synthetic medium, semi-synthetic medium	2012
Hep A (Havrix)	aluminum hydroxide, amino acid supplement, polysorbate 20, formalin, neomycin sulfate, MRC-5 cellular proteins	December 2013
Hep A (Vaqta)	amorphous aluminum hydroxyphosphate sulfate, bovine albumin, formaldehyde, neomycin, sodium borate, MRC-5 (human diploid) cells	February 2014
Hep B (Engerix-B)	aluminum hydroxide, yeast protein, phosphate buffers, sodium dihydrogen phosphate dihydrate	December 2013
Hep B (Recombivax)	yeast protein, soy peptone, dextrose, amino acids, mineral salts, potassium aluminum sulfate, amorphous aluminum hydroxyphosphate sulfate, formaldehyde, phosphate buffer	May 2014
Hep A/Hep B (Twinrix)	formalin, yeast protein, aluminum phosphate, aluminum hydroxide, amino acids, phosphate buffer, polysorbate 20, neomycin sulfate, MRC-5 human diploid cells	August 2012
Human Papillomavirus (HPV) (Cerverix)	vitamins, amino acids, lipids, mineral salts, aluminum hydroxide, sodium dihydrogen phosphate dehydrate, 3-O-desacyl-4' Monophosphoryl lipid A, insect cell, bacterial, and viral protein	November 2013
Human Papillomavirus (HPV) (Gardasil)	yeast protein, vitamins, amino acids, mineral salts, carbohydrates, amorphous aluminum hydroxyphosphate sulfate, L-histidine, polysorbate 80, sodium borate	June 2014
Human Papillomavirus (HPV) (Gardasil 9)	yeast protein, vitamins, amino acids, mineral salts, carbohydrates, amorphous aluminum hydroxyphosphate sulfate, L-histidine, polysorbate 80, sodium borate	December 2014
Influenza (Afluria)	beta-propiolactone, thimerosol (multi-dose vials only), monobasic sodium phosphate, dibasic sodium phosphate, monobasic potassium phosphate, potassium chloride, calcium chloride, sodium taurodeoxycholate, neomycin sulfate, polymyxin B, egg protein, sucrose	December 2013
Influenza (Agriflu)	egg proteins, formaldehyde, polysorbate 80, cetyltrimethylammonium bromide, neomycin sulfate, kanamycin, barium	2013
Influenza (Fluarix) Trivalent and Quadrivalent	octoxynol-10 (Triton X-) J-tocopheryl hydrogen succinate, polysorbate 80 (Tween 80), hydrocortisone, gentamicin sulfate, ovalbumin, formaldehyde, sodium deoxycholate, sucrose, phosphate buffer	June 2014

APPENDIX A (CONTINUED)

APPENDIX A *(Continued)*

Influenza (Flublok)	monobasic sodium phosphate, dibasic sodium phosphate, polysorbate 20, baculovirus and host cell proteins, baculovirus and cellular DNA, Triton X-100, lipids, vitamins, amino acids, mineral salts	March 2014
Influenza (Flucelvax)	Madin Darby Canine Kidney (MDCK) cell protein, MDCK cell DNA, SRO\VRUEDWH FHW\OWULPHWKO\DPPRQLXP EUR-PLGH ü-propiolactone, phosphate buffer	March 2014
Influenza (Fluvirin)	nonylphenol ethoxylate, thimerosal (multidose vial–trace only in prefilled syringe), polymyxin, neomycin, beta-propiolactone, egg proteins, phosphate buffer	February 2014
Influenza (Flulaval) Trivalent and Quadrivalent	thimerosal, formaldehyde, sodium deoxycholate, egg proteins, phosphate buffer	February 2013
Influenza (Fluzone: Standard (Trivalent and Quadrivalent), High-Dose, & Intradermal)	formaldehyde, octylphenol ethoxylate (Triton X-100), gelatin (standard trivalent formulation only), thimerosal (multi-dose vial only), egg protein, phosphate buffers, sucrose	2014
Influenza (FluMist) Quadrivalent	ethylene diamine tetraacetic acid (EDTA), monosodium glutamate, hydrolyzed porcine gelatin, arginine, sucrose, dibasic potassium phosphate, monobasic potassium phosphate, gentamicin sulfate, egg protein	July 2013
Japanese Encephalitis (Ixiaro)	aluminum hydroxide, Vero cells, protamine sulfate, formaldehyde, bovine serum albumin, sodium metabisulphite, sucrose	May 2013
Meningococcal (MCV4Menactra)	formaldehyde, phosphate buffers, Mueller Hinton agar, Watson Scherp media, Modified Mueller and Miller medium, detergent, alcohol, ammonium sulfate	April 2013
Meningococcal (MCV4Menveo)	formaldehyde, amino acids, yeast extract, Franz complete medium, CY medium	August 2013
Meningococcal (MPSV4Menomune)	thimerosal (multi-dose vial only), lactose, Mueller Hinton casein agar, Watson Scherp media, detergent, alcohol	April 2013
Meningococcal (MenB – Bexsero)	aluminum hydroxide, E. coli, histidine, sucrose, deoxycholate, kanomycin	2015

APPENDIX A (CONTINUED)

APPENDIX A *(Continued)*

Meningococcal (MenB – Trumenba)	polysorbate 80, histidine, E. coli, fermentation growth media	October 2015
MMR (MMR-II)	Medium 199 (vitamins, amino acids, fetal bovine serum, sucrose, glutamate), Minimum Essential Medium, phosphate, recombinant human albumin, neomycin, sorbitol, hydrolyzed gelatin, chick embryo cell culture, WI-38 human diploid lung fibroblasts	June 2014
MMRV (ProQuad)	sucrose, hydrolyzed gelatin, sorbitol, monosodium L-glutamate, sodium phosphate dibasic, human albumin, sodium bicarbonate, potassium phosphate monobasic, potassium chloride, potassium phosphate dibasic, neomycin, bovine calf serum, chick embryo cell culture, WI-38 human diploid lung fibroblasts, MRC-5 cells	March 2014
Pneumococcal (PCV13 – Prevnar 13)	casamino acids, yeast, ammonium sulfate, Polysorbate 80, succinate buffer, aluminum phosphate, soy peptone broth	January 2014
Pneumococcal (PPSV-23 – Pneumovax)	phenol	May 2014
Polio (IPV – Ipol)	2-phenoxyethanol, formaldehyde, neomycin, streptomycin, polymyxin B, monkey kidney cells, Eagle MEM modified medium, calf serum protein, Medium 199	May 2013
Rabies (Imovax)	Human albumin, neomycin sulfate, phenol red indicator, MRC-5 human diploid cells, beta-propriolactone	April 2013
Rabies (RabAvert)	ü-propiolactone, potassium glutamate, chicken protein, egg protein, neomycin, chlortetracycline, amphotericin B, human serum albumin, polygeline (processed bovine gelatin), sodium EDTA, bovine serum	March 2012
Rotavirus (RotaTeq)	sucrose, sodium citrate, sodium phosphate monobasic monohydrate, sodium hydroxide, polysorbate 80, cell culture media, fetal bovine serum, vero cells [DNA from porcine circoviruses (PCV) 1 and 2 has been detected in RotaTeq. PCV-1 and PCV-2 are not known to cause disease in humans.]	June 2013
Rotavirus (Rotarix)	amino acids, dextran, sorbitol, sucrose, calcium carbonate, xanthan, Dulbecco's Modified Eagle Medium (potassium chloride, magnesium sulfate, ferric (III) nitrate, sodium phosphate, sodium pyruvate, D-glucose, concentrated vitamin solution, L-cystine, L-tyrosine, amino acids solution, L-glutamine, calcium chloride, sodium hydrogenocarbonate, and phenol red) [Porcine circovirus type 1 (PCV-1) is present in Rotarix. PCV-1 is not known to cause disease in humans.]	May 2014
Smallpox (Vaccinia – ACAM2000)	human serum albumin, mannitol, neomycin, glycerin, polymyxin B, phenol, Vero cells, HEPES	September 2009

APPENDIX A *(Continued)*

Vaccine	Ingredients	Date
Td (Decavac)	aluminum potassium sulfate, peptone, formaldehyde, thimerosal, bovine muscle tissue (US sourced), Mueller and Miller medium, ammonium sulfate	March 2011
Td (Tenivac)	aluminum phosphate, formaldehyde, modified Mueller-Miller casamino acid medium without beef heart infusion, ammonium sulfate	April 2013
Td (Mass Biologics)	aluminum phosphate, formaldehyde, thimerosal (trace), ammonium phosphate, modified Mueller's media (containing bovine extracts)	February 2011
Tdap (Adacel)	aluminum phosphate, formaldehyde, glutaraldehyde, 2-phenoxyethanol, ammonium sulfate, Stainer-Scholte medium, dimethyl-beta-cyclodextrin, modified Mueller's growth medium, Mueller-Miller casamino acid medium (without beef heart infusion)	March 2014
Tdap (Boostrix)	formaldehyde, glutaraldehyde, aluminum hydroxide, polysorbate 80 (Tween 80), Latham medium derived from bovine casein, Fenton medium containing a bovine extract, Stainer-Scholte liquid medium	February 2013
Typhoid (inactivated – Typhim Vi)	hexadecyltrimethylammonium bromide, formaldehyde, phenol, polydimethylsiloxane, disodium phosphate, monosodium phosphate, semi-synthetic medium	March 2014
Typhoid (oral – Ty21a)	yeast extract, casein, dextrose, galactose, sucrose, ascorbic acid, amino acids, lactose, magnesium stearate, gelatin	September 2013
Varicella (Varivax)	sucrose, phosphate, glutamate, gelatin, monosodium L-glutamate, sodium phosphate dibasic, potassium phosphate monobasic, potassium chloride, sodium phosphate monobasic, potassium chloride, EDTA, residual components of MRC-5 cells including DNA and protein, neomycin, fetal bovine serum, human diploid cell cultures (WI-38), embryonic guinea pig cell cultures, human embryonic lung cultures	March 2014
Yellow Fever (YF-Vax)	sorbitol, gelatin, egg protein	May 2013
Zoster (Shingles – Zostavax)	sucrose, hydrolyzed porcine gelatin, monosodium L-glutamate, sodium phosphate dibasic, potassium phosphate monobasic, neomycin, potassium chloride, residual components of MRC-5 cells including DNA and protein, bovine calf serum	February 2014

APPENDIX B

APPENDIX B
Body fat percentage charts for men and women, based on age. Find your age range in the left column and scan across to locate your body fat percentage number. The shade denotes the range for lean, ideal, average, and above average. For a 34-year-old woman, with body fat percentage of 25.1, this is within the ideal range.

MEN'S BODY FAT PERCENTAGE CHART

AGE IN YEARS																
18-20	2.0	3.9	6.2	8.5	10.5	12.5	14.3	16.0	17.5	18.9	20.2	21.3	22.3	23.1	23.8	24.3	24.9
21-25	2.5	4.9	7.3	9.5	11.6	13.6	15.4	17.0	18.6	20.0	21.2	22.3	23.3	24.2	24.9	25.4	25.8
26-30	3.5	6.0	8.4	10.6	12.7	14.6	16.4	18.1	19.6	21.0	22.3	23.4	24.4	25.2	25.9	26.5	26.9
31-35	4.5	7.1	9.4	11.7	13.7	15.7	17.5	19.2	20.7	22.1	23.4	24.5	25.5	26.3	27.0	27.5	28.0
36-40	5.6	8.1	10.5	12.7	14.8	16.8	18.6	20.2	21.8	23.2	24.4	25.6	26.5	27.4	28.1	28.6	29.0
41-45	6.7	9.2	11.5	13.8	15.9	17.8	19.6	21.3	22.8	24.7	25.5	26.6	27.6	28.4	29.1	29.7	30.1
46-50	7.7	10.2	12.6	14.8	16.9	18.9	20.7	22.4	23.9	25.3	26.6	27.7	28.7	29.5	30.2	30.7	31.2
51-55	8.8	11.3	13.7	15.9	18.0	20.0	21.8	23.4	25.0	26.4	27.6	28.7	29.7	30.6	31.2	31.8	32.2
56+	9.9	12.4	14.7	17.0	19.1	21.0	22.8	24.5	26.0	27.4	28.7	29.8	30.8	31.6	32.3	32.9	33.3
	LEAN						IDEAL			AVERAGE				ABOVE AVERAGE		

WOMEN'S BODY FAT PERCENTAGE

AGE IN YEARS																
18-20	11.3	13.5	15.7	17.7	19.7	21.5	23.2	24.8	26.3	27.7	29.0	30.2	31.3	32.3	33.1	33.9	34.6
21-25	11.9	14.2	16.3	18.4	20.3	22.1	23.8	25.5	27.0	28.4	29.6	30.8	31.9	32.9	33.8	34.5	35.2
26-30	12.5	14.8	16.9	19.0	20.9	22.7	24.5	26.1	27.6	29.0	30.3	31.5	32.6	33.5	34.4	35.2	35.8
31-35	13.2	15.4	17.6	19.6	21.5	23.4	25.1	26.7	28.2	29.6	30.9	32.1	33.2	34.1	35.0	35.8	36.4
36-40	13.8	16.0	18.2	20.2	22.2	24.0	25.7	27.3	28.8	30.2	31.5	32.7	33.8	34.8	35.6	36.4	37.0
41-45	14.4	16.7	18.8	20.8	22.8	24.6	26.3	27.9	29.4	30.8	32.1	33.3	34.4	35.4	36.3	37.0	37.7
46-50	15.0	17.3	19.4	21.5	23.4	25.2	26.9	28.6	30.1	31.5	32.8	34.0	35.0	36.0	36.9	37.6	38.3
51-55	15.6	17.9	20.0	22.1	24.0	25.9	27.6	29.2	30.7	32.1	33.4	34.6	35.6	36.6	37.5	38.3	38.9
56+	16.3	18.5	20.7	22.7	24.6	26.5	28.2	29.8	31.3	32.7	34.0	35.2	36.3	37.2	38.1	38.9	39.5
	LEAN						IDEAL			AVERAGE				ABOVE AVERAGE		

APPENDIX C

APPENDIX C

BMI Chart values. Line up your weight with height and find the intersecting number. For a 180-pound man at 6'0" tall, the BMI is 24, and in the healthy range.

Weight lbs.	100	105	110	115	120	125	130	135	140	145	150	155	160	165	170	175	180	185	190	195	200	205	210	215
Height																								
5'0"	19	20	21	22	23	24	25	26	27	28	29	30	31	32	33	34	35	36	37	38	39	40	41	42
5'1"	18	19	20	21	22	23	24	25	26	27	28	29	30	31	32	33	34	35	36	36	37	38	39	40
5'2"	18	19	20	21	22	22	23	24	25	26	27	28	29	30	31	32	33	33	34	35	36	37	38	39
5'3"	17	18	19	20	21	22	23	24	24	25	26	27	28	29	30	31	32	32	33	34	35	36	37	38
5'4"	17	18	18	19	20	21	22	23	24	25	26	27	28	28	29	30	31	32	33	33	34	35	36	37
5'5"	16	17	18	19	20	21	21	22	23	24	25	26	27	27	28	29	30	31	32	32	33	34	35	35
5'6"	16	17	17	18	19	20	21	22	23	23	24	25	26	27	27	28	29	30	31	31	32	33	34	34
5'7"	15	16	17	18	18	19	20	21	22	22	23	24	25	26	26	27	28	29	29	30	31	32	33	33
5'8"	15	16	16	17	18	19	19	20	21	22	22	23	24	25	25	26	27	28	28	29	30	31	32	32
5'9"	14	15	16	17	17	18	19	20	20	21	22	23	23	24	25	25	26	27	28	28	29	30	31	31
5'10"	14	15	15	16	17	18	18	19	20	21	21	22	23	23	24	25	25	26	27	28	28	29	30	30
5'11"	14	14	15	16	17	17	18	19	19	20	21	21	22	23	23	24	25	25	26	27	28	28	29	30
6'0"	13	14	15	15	16	17	18	18	19	19	20	21	21	22	23	23	24	25	25	26	27	27	28	29
6'1"	13	13	14	15	15	16	17	17	18	19	19	20	21	21	22	23	23	24	25	25	26	27	27	28
6'2"	12	13	14	14	15	16	16	17	18	18	19	20	20	21	21	22	23	23	24	25	25	26	27	27
6'3"	12	13	13	14	15	15	16	17	17	18	18	19	20	20	21	21	22	23	23	24	25	25	26	26
6'4"	12	12	13	14	14	15	15	16	17	17	18	18	19	20	20	21	22	22	23	23	24	25	25	26

Underweight | Healthy | Overweight | Obese | Extremely Obese

APPENDIX D

The amount of fructose per serving of various fruits.

Fruit	Serving Size	Grams of Fructose
Limes	1 medium	0
Lemons	1 medium	0.6
Cranberries	1 cup	0.7
Prune	1 medium	1.2
Apricot	1 medium	1.3
Cantaloupe	1/8 medium	2.8
Raspberries	1 cup	3.0
Kiwifruit	1 medium	3.4
Blackberries	1 cup	3.5
Strawberries	1 cup	3.8
Cherries	1 cup	4.0
Pineapple	1 slice	4.0
Grapefruit	1/2 medium	4.3
Boysenberries	1 cup	4.6
Tangerine/Mandarin	1 medium	4.8
Peach	1 medium	6.1
Orange	1 medium	6.1
Papaya	1/2 medium	6.3
Honeydew	1/8 medium	6.7
Banana	1 medium	7.1
Blueberries	1 cup	7.4.
Apple	1 medium	9.5
Watermelon	1/16 medium	11.3
Pear	1 medium	11.8
Raisins	1/4 cup	12.3
Grapes (red/green)	1 cup	12.4
Mango	1/2 medium	16.2
Apricots	1 cup	16.4

ABOUT THE AUTHOR

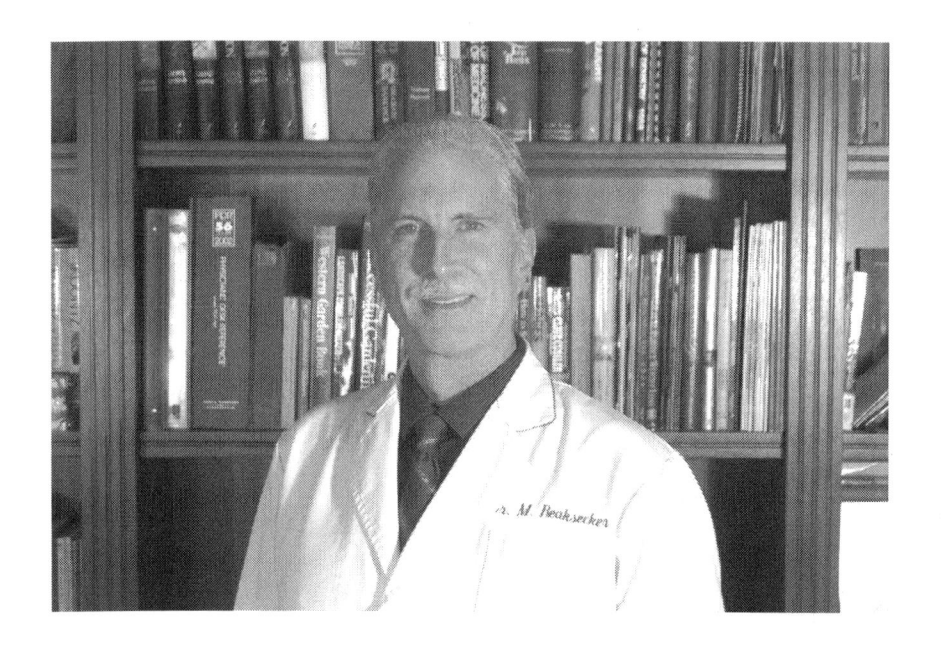

Mark Reaksecker, DMD is a graduate of the Oregon Health & Science University School of Dentistry and maintained a private dental practice for over 28 years. Throughout those years, he marveled at the complexity and capabilities of the human body with its ability to heal, even from adverse circumstances. The body is an amazing creation—the gift of life from God.

His in-depth study of nutrition and cancer, plus how they affect the human body, intensified the curiosity of how biology, physiology, and chemistry all play interactive roles. It took four years to research and two years to write this book, but it was a creation from his passion and the unending desire to learn.

Dr. Mark and his wife can be seen on the back cover. They try to epitomize the Garden of Eden Lifestyle by manifesting a living testimony and practice the procedures described herein.

During his free time, Dr. Mark volunteers as a member of the Royal Rosarians in Portland, Oregon. They are the official ambassadors for the city of Portland and travel the world planting roses. Portland is known as the city of roses with its beautiful rose garden overlooking Portland at Washington Park. The Rosarians can be seen on television every year marching in the Grand Floral Parade along the city streets of Portland the first weekend in June.

Dr. Mark appreciates traveling and photographing God's beautiful planet Earth. He enjoys skiing and scuba diving. Together, they have three grown children, two boys and one girl, but no grandchildren—yet. They reside in Oregon City, Oregon, which is southeast of Portland in the Willamette Valley.

To learn more, visit Dr. Mark's website at:

http://www.healthybodyhappylifebook.com

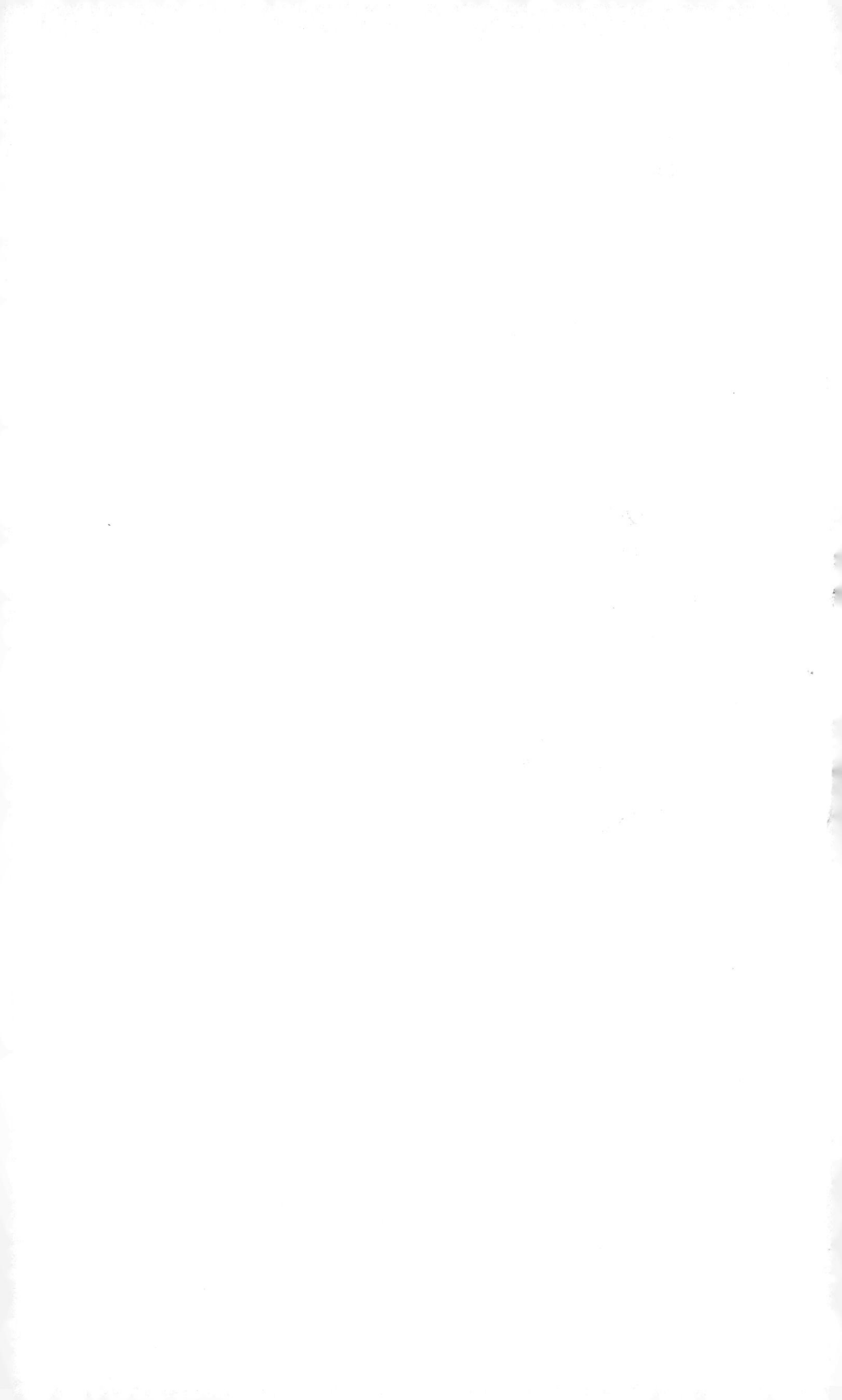

Made in the USA
San Bernardino, CA
17 June 2017